The Praeger Handbook of Acupuncture for Pain Management

The Praeger Handbook of Acupuncture for Pain Management

A Guide to How the "Magic Needles" Work

Jun Xu, MD, L.Ac

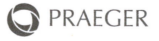

PRAEGER

AN IMPRINT OF ABC-CLIO, LLC
Santa Barbara, California • Denver, Colorado • Oxford, England

Library of Congress Cataloging-in-Publication Data

Xu, Jun, 1956– author.
    The Praeger handbook of acupuncture for pain management : a guide to how the "magic needles" work / Jun Xu.
        p. ; cm.
    Handbook of acupuncture for pain management
    Includes bibliographical references and index.
        ISBN 978-0-313-39701-1 (hardback : alk. paper) —
ISBN 978-0-313-39702-8 (EISBN)
    I. Title. II. Title: Handbook of acupuncture for pain management.
[DNLM: 1. Acupuncture Therapy—methods—Case Reports.
2. Pain Management—Case Reports. WB 369]
    RM184
    615.8'92—dc23   2014017828

ISBN: 978-0-313-39701-1
EISBN: 978-0-313-39702-8

18 17 16 15 14   1 2 3 4 5

This book is also available on the World Wide Web as an eBook.
Visit www.abc-clio.com for details.

Praeger
An Imprint of ABC-CLIO, LLC

ABC-CLIO, LLC
130 Cremona Drive, P.O. Box 1911
Santa Barbara, California 93116-1911

This book is printed on acid-free paper ∞

Manufactured in the United States of America

This book discusses treatments (including types of medication and mental health therapies), diagnostic tests for various symptoms and mental health disorders, and organizations. The authors have made every effort to present accurate and up-to-date information. However, the information in this book is not intended to recommend or endorse particular treatments or organizations, or substitute for the care or medical advice of a qualified health professional, or used to alter any medical therapy without a medical doctor's advice. Specific situations may require specific therapeutic approaches not included in this book. For those reasons, we recommend that readers follow the advice of qualified health care professionals directly involved in their care. Readers who suspect they may have specific medical problems should consult a physician about any suggestions made in this book.

Contents

Acknowledgments

This is my second book about the *magic needles*. I feel very much in debt to the following people—without their support, this book would never have reached my readers.

Caroline Hutton, my agent, whose encouragement gave me the strength to continue my writing.

Roberta Waddell, my editor, who made endless efforts to improve my manuscript and make it more readable to my lay audience.

Robert Blizzard, DPT, my colleague and a doctor of physical therapy, who provided much of the information on physical therapy.

Cathy Snyder-Kovacs, my art editor, who helped me modify entire figures. Her talent and devotion gave me the strength to finish this book.

Melanie Chow, who helped me reshape my draft when she was an English student at Brown University.

My patients. Since all the cases have come from my clinical practice, I could not have written any of the case studies without their support and active participation. Their questions are always fascinating and thought-provoking.

Hong Su, CMD, my wife, a licensed acupuncturist, who gave me the motivation to finish my second book.

Debbie Carvalko, my editor at Praeger, who kept me on the straight and narrow during the writing. Her patience motivated me to work hard for this book.

ACUPUNCTURE'S IMPORTANCE

Acupuncture releases a natural energy (qi) that can alleviate even long-standing health problems. Pain-free acupuncture is, therefore, an ideal treatment for a broad spectrum of painful conditions, from the top of the head all the way down through the body to the toes.

Unlike acupressure, a self-help method, acupuncture requires a practitioner, so you may want to show the acupuncturist you visit the chapters here that correspond to your pain condition. The valuable information in this book includes the techniques involved in a wide variety of the many painful conditions that acupuncture so successfully treats. At the end of each chapter, there are tips for both acupuncturists and patients that can provide additional help and increase the personal experience.

Introduction

Acupuncture is a skillful method of inserting one or more needles into specific anatomic points in the body in order to induce an energy flow that can heal and modify illness. For thousands of years in China, many physicians have tried to summarize their experiences, hoping to make the public understand their theory. Many books on acupuncture have been written, but their complex terminology is often difficult to understand, and most of them elaborate on Chinese medicine without giving any specific explanations for the theories and methods of traditional Chinese medicine (TCM).

Since TCM was introduced into the West in the late 17th century, many Western physicians have tried to understand its theories that were originally written in the deep and difficult Chinese language, and have tried to translate the TCM theory into Western languages. After learning some of the TCM procedures, many of these doctors go on to practice the method with great success. For many others, however, this is not the case, for a number of reasons. First, there is the language barrier and the difference in backgrounds between practitioners and patients in China and those in Western countries; then there is the huge difference between Western medicine and TCM. Many acupuncture and other TCM treatments for diseases and illnesses are not very well understood by practitioners in the West. Because many of them, and many of their patients, do not understand the TCM theory and language, they cannot clearly explain this difficult theory and practice in their Western languages. In addition, for hundreds of years, Western medicine has been predominant in the West, to the exclusion of other systems, with the end result that many of these doctors simply do not believe in the efficacy of TCM. This is, as noted, partially because of the language barrier, but it is also because there is a lack of scientific research available on acupuncture and TCM (though this is changing).

Even with the huge differences between TCM and Western medicine, the ultimate goal of both is, and has always been, the same—to treat illness and alleviate a patient's aches and pains. That is the common ground between both medical systems.

The first part of the book concerns information and theories about acupuncture, followed by chapters on theories of TCM, including yin and yang, the five elements, the zang-fu organs, and the meridians.

Using the terminology of Western medicine, the balance of the book discusses 30 case histories, beginning at the head and ending at the foot, with a focus on painful conditions that acupuncture can alleviate. It outlines brief physical examinations to determine the symptoms and causes of the condition, and to diagnose it in relation to both Western and TCM procedures. Following the section on treatments in Western medicine, each case ends with treatments in TCM/acupuncture, giving simple explanations of the basic TCM theory for each specific condition and then listing the locations of the acupuncture points, accompanied by illustrations and/or diagrams. The reason for this detailed information is threefold.

1. To know where the points are and be able to use them for self-massage to help alleviate your ailment.
2. To be able to discuss the selection of the points in your treatment with your acupuncturist.
3. To understand your illness within the dual frameworks of both Western and TCMs.

As an acupuncturist, you can use this book for the following:

1. To understand some concepts of Western medicine, including anatomy, physiology, and pathology.
2. To learn the acupuncture points and their selection. In easily understandable language, this book explains various medical conditions in both Western and TCM. It does not matter whether you have a background in Western medicine or one in TCM; you can learn from your reading.

This book has been written with you, the reader, in mind. I believe you will enjoy reading it.

PART ONE

Acupuncture Information and Theories

1

A Brief History
of Acupuncture

For thousands of years, ancient people used traditional medicine for the health of the mind, the body, and the spirit; thus acupuncture may be almost as old as mankind itself. Millennia before the birth of Christ, as far back as the Stone Age, medical practitioners in China were practicing a rudimentary form of acupuncture, using pointed stone *needles* to stimulate certain points in the human body. Needles of this period were also made of sharpened ivory from the bones and tusks of slaughtered beasts used for food and skins, and were known as *bian shi.*

Acupuncture was believed to alleviate, or even cure, all manner and conditions of illnesses affecting the body, mind, and spirit. The needles were placed along the meridians of the human body and were believed to encourage the proper flow of *qi* (pronounced *chee*). This term is not translatable but can be understood as the life force, or energy, which keeps the body functioning. There are approximately 400 commonly used acupuncture points found along the 12 major meridians and the other minor meridians in the body.

Many ancient civilizations believed in this life energy (qi) that affected the mind as well as the body and also flowed into the physical world beyond.

This release of energy is thought to stimulate different life systems, including the immune system, and to produce necessary qi and blood in all components of the body, keeping all in perfect balance and harmony. These two factors, balance and harmony, encompass the elements that make up the earth and everything in it, including the human body. Current research indicates that all energy on the earth originated from the sun, and it strongly supports this theory of energy flowing throughout and beyond the human body.

The earliest known medical book, called *Yellow Emperor's Canon of Medicine* (*Huang Di Nei Jing* in Chinese) and published in two volumes, written in China by various people involved with medicine, took almost 200 years to complete (ca. 500 BC–ca. 300 BC), and it contains all the known facts about healing arts known up to that time. It was widely accepted as *the* definitive work encompassing all the tenets of medicine, including acupuncture. (Other topics it covered were yin-yang, the five elements, diagnostic methods, the major and lesser meridians, and Chinese herbs.)

Subsequently, thousands of books on the subject of traditional Chinese medicine (TCM) were published, and they dealt mainly with acupuncture and moxibustion. Additionally, in early Chinese art, there are examples of the acupuncture points imposed on the human figure.

Chinese acupuncture spread east to Korea, Japan, Vietnam, and other Asian countries, and later made its way to Europe. *Iceman,* a mummified human believed to be 5,000 years old, was discovered in Italy and is now displayed in a museum in Bolzano, Italy. It exhibits tattoos on its body, some of which have been identified as corresponding to the classic points of Chinese acupuncture, leading scholars to surmise that acupuncture was used in Europe 3,000 years before the birth of Christ.

It is believed that, initially, needles used for acupuncture were placed at

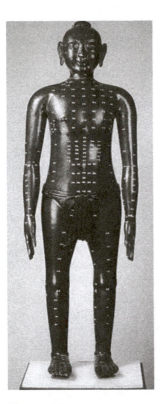

random points in the human body. After centuries of observation as to which points were more successful in treating a particular illness, what emerged was the current model of acupuncture points that follow along the various major and minor meridians believed to run through the human body. This data was collected and compiled in 1026 by Wang Wei-ye, who wrote the *Illustrated Manual on the Points for Acupuncture and Moxibustion as Found on the Bronze Figure,* published in 1027, which became the most important book on the subject; over the next 300 years, this work evolved into the approximately 400 acupuncture points frequently used today. The author also made a *bronze human body model,* which depicted 354 points used for acupuncture and gave detailed drawings of their ·exact placement on the human body (see Figure 1.1).

Acupuncture continued to be practiced throughout China for approximately the next 600 years, but with the coming of the Qing dynasty (1644–1911), the top doctors of the time were offering herbal remedies more often than acupuncture. Even so, acupuncture was tremendously developed in the Qing dynasty as well.

Figure 1.1

There were many wars in China during the first 50 years of the 20th century. In this time, except for some small schools established by acupuncturists, no medical schools sponsored by the government officially taught acupuncture and TCM. This changed in 1949, however, because the Chinese government leaders wished to elevate all things Chinese. They returned acupuncture to its place in the hierarchy of medicine and proposed to make traditional medicine, as practiced over the centuries, again popular, once again having it originate in China as it had centuries before. Therefore, hospitals and medical schools once more began teaching acupuncture to their students, and the discipline has prevailed to this day.

Acupuncture slowly crossed the Atlantic Ocean and only became known after the summer of 1971, when an American journalist, James Reston of the *New York Times,* had an emergency appendectomy while on assignment in China. Two nights after the operation, he was experiencing some abdominal discomfort (bloating, abdominal pain, and stomachache), and he was treated by the acupuncturist, Dr. Li Chang-Yuan, while in the hospital. Reston wrote that the acupuncture needles "inserted in the outer part of my right elbow and below my knees . . . sent ripples of pain racing through my limbs and, at least, had the effect of diverting attention from the distress in my stomach. Meanwhile Dr. Li lit two pieces of an herb called Ai, which looked like the burning stumps of a broken cheap cigar, and held them close to my abdomen while occasionally twirling the needles into action." This article brought acupuncture to the United States.[1]

While earlier acupuncture needles must have been extremely primitive, and probably painful as well, today's disposable needles are made of stainless steel, no thicker than a hair shaft. Most people feel nothing at all when the needles are inserted; a few feel minimum pain, which passes as the needles proceed to do their work.

The use of herbs also plays an important role in TCM. The development and use of a multitude of herbs probably go back as far as the origins of acupuncture, as early man discovered that certain plants found locally helped alleviate some of the suffering experienced at the time. This is a vast subject and will be covered in a future volume.

2

The Mechanism of Acupuncture

EASTERN EXPLANATION

The human body has 14 meridians that are like a circulating net around the body, and these meridians connect all major organs and body surfaces. The life energy called qi (chee) that flows through this net can be influenced and balanced by stimulating specific points on the body's surface. According to Chinese medical theory, illness arises when the cyclical flow of qi in the meridians is blocked or becomes unbalanced. By inserting needles at certain points along the 14 meridians, accompanied by specific stimulation or manipulation, the acupuncture treatment will have the following functions:

1. *Adjusting.* Acupuncture treatment induces a smooth flow of energy in the body, and yin and yang keep an energy balance in the entire body.
2. *Expelling the negative energy* from the internal organs. By enhancing the positive energy, the illness energy will be expelled, which will maintain a balance in the body.
3. *Improving the circulation of energy* along the 14 meridians. The distal parts of the body also need energy circulation, and acupuncture treatment can facilitate this.
4. *Treating the root of the illness* by recovering the function of internal organs. Because many illnesses originate from unbalanced internal organs, after they are balanced, the root of the illness can then be searched out and specifically treated.

WESTERN EXPLANATION

Acupuncture points are areas of designated electrical sensitivity. Inserting needles at these points stimulates various sensory receptors that, in turn, stimulate nerves that transmit impulses to the brain's surface and different pathway systems, which will subsequently trigger many electro-physiological, biophysiological, and biochemical changes.

THE MELZACK/WALL THEORY OF PAIN

Ronald Melzack and P. D. Wall proposed the gate-control theory in 1962. In their famous articles, they indicated that pain perception is mediated by the cooperation of excitation and inhibition in pain pathways and that it is not simply a direct response to the stimulation of pain fibers.

The perception of pain can be altered through inhibitory action on the pain pathway; therefore, the feeling of pain can be reduced or changed. In other words, there is a gate on the pain pathway, where the pain sensation can be switched on or off through various methods—mechanically, pharmacologically, physically, physiologically, and psychologically.[1]

Three neuropathways located in the spinal cord act to influence the perception of pain. They are the substantia gelatinosa in the dorsal horn, the dorsal column fibers, and the central transmission cells, which are composed of large and small fibers.[2]

Stimulation of the large-diameter fibers inhibits the transmission of pain, thus *closing the gate*. When the gate is closed, signals from small-diameter pain fibers will be switched off to reduce pain perception. When smaller fibers are stimulated, however, the gate is opened and pain signals excite dorsal horn transmission cells, which enhance the perception of pain.

In 1976, the gate-control theory was used to explain the mechanisms of acupuncture. Melzack suggested that acupuncture acts on the reticular formation in the brain stem to alter the pain pathway.[3]

Many studies have supported this theory about the mechanisms of acupuncture. Melzack's idea led to the theory of pain-gating being controlled centrally, and this led to the proposition that pain gets blockaded at the brain, not at the spinal cord or the periphery, through the release of natural painkillers in the brain (endogenous opioids), and neurohormones such as endorphins and naturally occurring morphines (enkephalins).[4, 5]

3

Diseases Where Acupuncture Can Be Helpful

There are a number of surveys and much data indicating that acupuncture has been used for treatment of many diseases in the United States.

CALIFORNIA STATE ACUPUNCTURE COMMITTEE SURVEY

In 1996, an occupational survey was conducted under contract to the California State Acupuncture Committee to update the content of the California Acupuncture Licensing Exam. This survey identified well over 100 conditions or categories of conditions treated, and the following is a list of the top 25 conditions that licensed acupuncturists treated.[1]

Twenty-Five Conditions Commonly Treated by Acupuncture

- Anxiety and depression
- Arthritis, tendonitis, and joint pain
- Asthma and allergies
- Auto injuries
- Bladder and kidney infections
- Cardiac palpitations (irregular heartbeat)
- Chronic fatigue syndrome
- Common cold and influenza
- Degenerative disc disorders
- Diet, nutrition, and weight control
- Fibromyalgia
- Headaches and migraines
- Hypertension (high blood pressure)
- Indigestion, gas, bloating, and constipation
- Insomnia
- Menopause symptoms
- Musculoskeletal pain
- Nausea
- Orthopedic conditions
- Pain—other kinds
- PMS and menstrual irregularity
- Sports injuries
- Tension/stress syndromes
- Tinnitus
- Work injuries

MARYLAND ACUPUNCTURE SOCIETY—PATIENT SATISFACTION SURVEY

Thirteen Conditions Commonly and Effectively Treated by Acupuncture

The Maryland Acupuncture Society contracted for a patient survey to be conducted in 1999, with the results being published in January 2000. The Patient Satisfaction Survey—Final Report lists the 13 most common conditions for which patients sought treatment from an acupuncturist. Over 80 percent of the respondents found these treatments to be either very effective or moderately effective.

- Allergies
- Arthritis
- Asthma
- Back pain
- Depression/mood disorders
- Fatigue/energy
- Female concerns
- Gastrointestinal problems
- Headaches
- Health/wholeness
- Migraine headaches
- Musculoskeletal pain
- Stress/tension

WORLD HEALTH ORGANIZATION (WHO) EXPERTS' REPORT ON ACUPUNCTURE

Acupuncture Recognized as Therapeutic Tool for Many Types of Illness

In 2003, experts from the WHO pointed out the diseases and disorders that can be treated with acupuncture.[2]

1. This is a list of the diseases, symptoms, or conditions for which acupuncture has proved—through controlled trials—to be an effective treatment.

   - Adverse reactions to radiotherapy and/or chemotherapy
   - Allergic rhinitis (including hay fever)
   - Biliary colic
   - Correction of malposition of fetus
   - Depression (including depressive neurosis and depression following stroke)
   - Dysentery, acute bacillary
   - Dysmenorrhoea, primary
   - Epigastralgia, acute (in peptic ulcer, acute and chronic gastritis, and gastrospasm)
   - Facial pain (including craniomandibular disorders)

- Headache
- Hypertension, essential
- Hypotension, primary
- Induction of labor
- Knee pain
- Leukopenia
- Low back pain
- Morning sickness
- Nausea and vomiting
- Neck pain
- Pain in dentistry (including dental pain and temporomandibular dysfunction)
- Periarthritis of shoulder
- Postoperative pain
- Renal colic
- Rheumatoid arthritis
- Sciatica
- Sprain
- Stroke
- Tennis elbow

2. Diseases, symptoms, or conditions for which the therapeutic effect of acupuncture has been shown but for which further proof is needed.

- Abdominal pain (in acute gastroenteritis or due to gastrointestinal spasm)
- Acne vulgaris
- Alcohol dependence and detoxification
- Bell's palsy
- Bronchial asthma
- Cancer pain
- Cardiac neurosis
- Cholecystitis, chronic, with acute exacerbation
- Cholelithiasis
- Competition stress syndrome
- Craniocerebral injury, closed
- Diabetes mellitus, non-insulin-dependent
- Earache
- Epidemic hemorrhagic fever
- Epistaxis, simple (without generalized or local disease)
- Eye pain due to subconjunctival injection
- Female infertility
- Facial spasm
- Female urethral syndrome
- Fibromyalgia and fasciitis
- Gastrokinetic disturbance
- Gouty arthritis
- Hepatitis B virus carrier status
- Herpes zoster (human-alpha-herpesvirus 3)
- Hyperlipaemia
- Hypo-ovarianism
- Insomnia
- Labor pain
- Lactation, deficiency
- Male sexual dysfunction, non-organic
- Ménière's disease
- Neuralgia, post-herpetic
- Neurodermatitis
- Obesity
- Opium, cocaine, and heroin dependence
- Osteoarthritis
- Pain due to endoscopic examination
- Pain in thromboangiitis obliterans

- Polycystic ovary syndrome (Stein–Leventhal syndrome)
- Postextubation in children
- Postoperative convalescence
- Premenstrual syndrome
- Prostatitis, chronic
- Pruritus
- Radicular and pseudoradicular pain syndrome
- Raynaud's syndrome, primary
- Recurrent lower urinary tract infection
- Reflex sympathetic dystrophy
- Retention of urine, traumatic
- Schizophrenia
- Sialism, drug-induced
- Sjögren's syndrome
- Sore throat (including tonsillitis)
- Spinal pain, acute
- Stiff neck
- Temporomandibular joint dysfunction
- Tietze syndrome
- Tobacco dependence
- Tourette syndrome
- Ulcerative colitis, chronic
- Urolithiasis
- Vascular dementia
- Whooping cough (pertussis)

3. Diseases, symptoms, or conditions for which there are only individual controlled trials reporting some therapeutic effects, but for which acupuncture is worth trying because treatment by conventional and other therapies is difficult.

- Chloasma
- Choroidopathy, central serous
- Color blindness
- Deafness
- Hypophrenia
- Irritable bowel syndrome
- Neuropathic bladder in spinal cord injury
- Pulmonary heart disease, chronic
- Small airway obstruction

4. Diseases, symptoms, or conditions for which acupuncture may be tried, provided the practitioner has special modern medical knowledge and adequate monitoring equipment.

- Breathlessness in chronic obstructive pulmonary disease
- Coma
- Convulsions in infants
- Coronary heart disease (angina pectoris)
- Diarrhea in infants and young children
- Encephalitis, viral, in children, late stage
- Paralysis, progressive bulbar and pseudobulbar

Based on the theory of traditional Chinese medicine, many diseases can be treated by acupuncture through the mechanism of adjusting the yin-yang balance, that is, inducing the energy of the human body to treat the illness. Therefore, it is reasonable to try acupuncture treatment as your personal choice. However, it is wise to consult your physician about any possible long-term effects before you try acupuncture. For some diseases, such as cancer and acute infectious diseases, I suggest you go to your primary physician before you go to a general acupuncturist.

4

The Advance of Acupuncture Research

The National Institutes of Health has not met since 1997 to review any new medical research done in the last 17 years. This chapter, therefore, reviews the accumulated research and discusses recently published findings regarding the uses of acupuncture and the many illnesses it can alleviate or cure.[1]

Acupuncture first came to the American consciousness in 1971 after Richard Nixon visited China. After that, more and more Americans came to appreciate the benefits of acupuncture treatment and traditional Chinese medicine because it is simple, is effective, and has almost no side effects. In a 2007 survey, 3.2 million Americans had had acupuncture treatments in the previous year—up from 2.1 million in 2001, according to the National Center for Complementary and Alternative Medicine. Showing more and more scientific evidence of the beneficial results of acupuncture, the treatment encompassed all types of Americans, from such big cities as New York and San Francisco to U.S. military bases in Iraq and Afghanistan.[2]

THE GATE-CONTROL THEORY OF PAIN

As early as 1962, Drs. Ronald Melzack and Patrick D. Wall suggested the gate-control theory of pain. They believed that pain perception and gate control existed within the dorsal horn of the spinal cord, that small nerve fibers were pain receptors and transmit sharp pain, and that large nerve fibers were normal receptors and send dull pain, as well as temperature sensations, with tracts to the brain. After the process of inhibitory interneurons, that is, the neurons, located between the brain and body, try to reduce the pain sensation transmitted to the brain by different processes, most pain becomes bearable to the human body. In other

words, various methods, such as mechanical, pharmacological, physiological, and physiological, can inhibit or block the pain pathway, lessening
or eliminating the perception of pain.

After studying the mechanism of acupuncture, Dr. Melzack suggested
that by inserting needles into certain points of the body, the energy (qi)
might alter the pain perception in the brain, change the quality and quan-
tity of pain impulse, and actually reduce the sensation of pain.

Further studies indicated that pain is blocked at the brain by the release
of endogenous opioids and neurohormones, such as endorphins and enkephalins (naturally occurring morphines).[3, 4, 5]

CONTEMPORARY ACUPUNCTURE MODEL—
NEUROHORMONAL THEORY

Neurohormonal theory indicates that the central neurotransmitters, such
as endorphin levels, might play a very important role in their regulation
in many levels of the brain along the pain pathway. Acupuncture may increase secretion after deqi (a composite of unique sensations—the person
will feel heaviness and dull pain after the needles inserted in the body are
twisted). However, if the endorphin receptors are blocked by medications,
such as Naloxone, the pain-reducing effects of acupuncture will be completely blocked.[6, 7]

Scientists from the Martinos Center for Biomedical Imaging at
Massachusetts General Hospital in Boston have recently used a functional MRI to study the effects of acupuncture on the BOLD (blood-
oxygen-level dependence) response and the functional connectivity of
the human brain. Results demonstrate that acupuncture affects a network
of systems in the brain, including decreasing activity in the limbic system. This is the emotional part of the brain, and it typically lights up in
various parts when the brain is at rest. Their studies support the neurohormonal theory.[8, 9, 10]

RECENT PROGRESS IN RESEARCHING CONDITIONS
SUITABLE FOR ACUPUNCTURE TREATMENT

Acupuncture Treatment for Chronic Pain

Chronic pain is a major indication for acupuncture. Individual data meta-
analyses were conducted using data from 25 of 31 eligible randomized
controlled trials (RCTs), with a total of 17,922 patients analyzed.

In the primary analysis, including all eligible RCTs, results showed
that acupuncture was superior to both sham (sham acupuncture is an

experimental design of putting a guiding tube on the acupuncture point without inserting a needle) and no-acupuncture control for each pain condition. After exclusion of an outlying set of RCTs that strongly favored acupuncture, the effects were similar across pain conditions.

The conclusion reached was that acupuncture is effective for the treatment of chronic pain and is therefore a reasonable referral option. Significant differences between true and sham acupuncture indicate that acupuncture is more effective than the placebo.[11]

Acupuncture Treatment for Plantar Fasciitis (Heel Pain)

Many people experience plantar fasciitis—heel pain (heel spur). Five RCTs and three non-randomized comparative studies were included in high-quality studies that reported significant benefits. In one, acupuncture was associated with significant improvement in pain and function when combined with standard treatment (including nonsteroidal anti-inflammatory drugs). In another, acupuncture point PC7 improved pain and pressure-pain threshold significantly more than acupuncture point LI4.

This is comparable to the evidence available for conventionally used interventions, such as stretching, night splints, or dexamethasone. Therefore, acupuncture should be considered in recommendations for the management of patients with Plantar Fasciitis.[12]

Acupuncture Treatment for Irritable Bowel Syndrome

Irritable bowel syndrome (IBS) is an illness characterized by alternate constipation and diarrhea without an obvious cause, and there is no effective treatment in Western medicine. Recently, a study was conducted on 233 people in England who had IBS with an average duration of 13 years; 116 of them were offered 10 weekly individualized acupuncture sessions plus Western medicine's usual care, including stool softener and anti-acid reflexes, and 117 of them continued with Western medicine's usual care alone. At three months, the groups showed a statistically significant difference, favoring acupuncture with a significant reduction in the severity of IBS symptoms.

The conclusion is that acupuncture for IBS provided an additional benefit over Western medicine's usual care alone, and the magnitude of the effect was sustained over the longer term. Acupuncture should be considered as a treatment option to be offered in primary care alongside other evidence-based treatments.[13]

Acupuncture Treatment to Reduce the Side Effects of Chemotherapy for People with Cancer

There are many studies that showed acupuncture can reduce the side effects of chemotherapy and radiotherapy for those with cancer, the main symptoms of which are nausea, vomiting, pain and fatigue, depression, shortness of breath, dry skin, and hot flashes.[14]

- Post-chemotherapy. Eleven trials of 1,247 cancer patients were studied collectively, to demonstrate the efficacy of acupuncture treatments of both acute and delayed chemotherapy-induced nausea and vomiting. One study showed that acupuncture treatment by inserting needles or self-administered acupressure in specific points is an effective method of reducing the symptoms of nausea and vomiting.[15]
- Postoperative nausea and vomiting. For 3,347 postoperative subjects in 26 trials, acupuncture point P6 was found to be very effective in reducing nausea and vomiting postoperatively. Manipulating the needles, either manually or by electronic stimulation, can enhance the effects.[16]

Acupuncture Treatment for Carpal Tunnel Syndrome (CTS)

The mainstream methods of noninvasive treatment for CTS are used in three ways to relieve the symptoms.

1. Orally, take two weeks of prednisolone, 20 mg daily, followed by two weeks of prednisolone, 10 mg daily;
2. Utilize a night splint; and
3. Administer acupuncture for four weeks, with two sessions per week.

A study from Taiwan concludes that short-term acupuncture treatment is as effective as short-term low-dose prednisolone for mild-to-moderate CTS. For those who have an intolerance or contraindication for oral steroids, or for those who do not opt for early surgery, acupuncture treatment provides an alternative choice.[17]

Another study from Thailand showed electro-acupuncture was as effective as night splinting with respect to overall symptoms and functions in mild-to-moderate CTS. However, pain was reduced more by electro-acupuncture than by night splinting.[18]

Acupuncture Treatment for Knee and Hip Pain

Of 490 potentially relevant articles, 14 RCTs involving 3,835 patients were included in the meta-analysis from July to October 2011. The conclusion was that acupuncture provided significantly better relief from osteoarthritis (OA) pain in the knee and a larger improvement in function than sham acupuncture, standard Western medicine's treatment, or waiting for further treatment.[19]

Selfe et al. showed the evidence of 10 trials representing 1,456 participants who met the inclusion criteria and were analyzed. These studies provide evidence that acupuncture is an effective treatment for pain and physical dysfunction associated with OA of the knee.[20]

There was a study of 3,633 Germans with severe hip pain who were treated with acupuncture. In an RCT, those with chronic pain due to OA of the knee or hip were randomly allocated to undergo up to 15 sessions of acupuncture in a three-month period, or to be a control group receiving no acupuncture. Another group of patients who did not consent to randomization underwent acupuncture treatment. All patients received the usual Western treatments, such as pain medicine, physical therapy, or rest, in addition to the study's treatment. Results of the treatment were compiled over a period of six months, and it was found that the changes in outcome in non-randomized patients were comparable with those in randomized patients who received acupuncture. These results indicate that acupuncture plus routine care is associated with a marked clinical improvement in those with chronic OA-associated pain of the knee or hip.[21]

Acupuncture Treatment for Impotence

Ninety patients with premature ejaculation referred to the urology clinic at a tertiary training and research hospital in Turkey were included in an RCT and randomly assigned into paroxetine, acupuncture, and placebo groups. Intra-vaginal ejaculation latency times were significantly prolonged after using paroxetine 20 mg/day, plus acupuncture treatment twice a week over a four-week period. Although less effective than daily paroxetine, acupuncture alone had a significantly stronger ejaculation-delaying effect than the placebo.[22]

Acupuncture Treatment for Infertility

The following are two famous studies for acupuncture treatment of infertility in women.

Two hundred twenty-five infertile women undergoing in vitro fertilization (IVF) in Germany were divided into two groups—group one with traditional luteal-phase acupuncture, and group two with sham acupuncture. The real acupuncture group had significantly higher clinical pregnancy and ongoing pregnancy rates (33.6% and 28.4%, respectively) than the sham acupuncture group (15.6% and 13.8%). These results indicated that acupuncture had significantly positive results on the outcome of IVF.[23]

A similar study, on a larger scale, was performed in China, with 1,366 women undergoing IVF using the same methods. This study completely reaffirmed the preceding results.[24]

Acupuncture for Low Back Pain

There are a number of studies that confirm the effectiveness of acupuncture treatment for low back pain (LBP).

In a multicenter, a randomized, patient-assessor blind, sham-controlled clinical trial was performed in Korea. One hundred thirty adults aged 18 to 65 who had non-specific LBP lasting for at least the prior three months participated. The results of this study suggest that acupuncture treatment shows better effects on the reduction of the pain intensity from LBP than sham control in participants with chronic LBP.[25]

In another study, a total of 159 people were treated in the acupuncture-offer arm and 80 in the usual-care arm. Offered acupuncture as an alternative to usual care, all 159 of these people chose to receive acupuncture, and received an average of eight acupuncture treatments within the trial.

The results showed that traditional acupuncture care delivered in a primary care setting was safe and acceptable to those with nonspecific LBP. Acupuncture care and usual care were both associated with clinically significant improvement at 12- and 24-month follow-ups. At a 24-month follow-up, however, acupuncture care was significantly more effective in reducing bodily pain than usual care. No benefits relating to function or disability were identified. General physicians referral to a service providing traditional acupuncture care offers a cost-effective intervention for reducing LBP over a two-year period.[26]

Acupuncture for Neck Pain

In total, 190 test subjects were recruited and 178 of them (88 in the study group and 90 in the control group) completed the intervention and follow-up assessment. The conclusion was that compared to the control group, traditional acupuncture was able to relieve the pain intensity and improve the quality of daily life, with a relative long-term clinical efficacy in those with chronic neck pain.[27]

Acupuncture for Shoulder Pain

The German randomized acupuncture trial for chronic shoulder pain (GRASP) was composed of 424 outpatients with chronic shoulder pain (CSP) who were randomly assigned to receive Chinese acupuncture (verum), sham acupuncture (sham), or conventional conservative orthopedic treatment. Which type of treatment they were to receive was not known to the subjects who were treated by 31 office-based orthopedists trained in acupuncture. All of them received 15 treatments over a six-week period. Descriptive statistics showed greater improvement of shoulder mobility (abduction and arm-above-head test) for the verum group versus the control group, both immediately after treatment and again after three months. The trial indicated that Chinese acupuncture is an effective alternative to conventional orthopedic treatment for CSP.[28]

5

The Choice of Acupuncturists

There are many acupuncturists in the United States. If you are considering acupuncture, do the same things you would in choosing a doctor.

- Ask people around for recommendations.
- Go to the government website to check the practitioner's training and credentials.

There are four types of acupuncturists practicing in the United States. Two groups are MD acupuncturists, and two are non-physician acupuncturists.

MD ACUPUNCTURISTS

1. Many licensed MD physicians in the United States actually graduated from Chinese medical schools, where they were trained in both Western medicine and Chinese acupuncture. These physicians are the best-trained group of acupuncturists. You should trust their ability to perform diagnosis and treatment for your illness, as long as they also have American MD license, which indicates that they received MD training in the United States.

2. Licensed MD physicians with regular acupuncture training from the United States. Many US licensed MD Physicians went to the UCLA School of Medicine and received a 300-hour acupuncture course that has been taught since 1983. About 6,000 American-licensed physicians received their certificates to practice acupuncture in the United States. These physician acupuncturists have strong training in Western medicine and a sound basic training in acupuncture. They also organize many conferences and provide an acupuncture subspecialty for physicians. They have earned the

reputation of conscientiously accomplishing the goal of creating clinically competent physician acupuncturists who can integrate acupuncture with conventional medicine. For more information, visit their website at http://www.cme.ucla.edu/courses.

Their graduates then formed the American Academy of Medical Acupuncture (AAMA). Their website—http://www.medicalacupuncture .org/aama_marf/aama.html lists—AAMA board-certified physician acupuncturists in your state.

NON-PHYSICIAN ACUPUNCTURISTS

1. For acupuncturists trained in the United States, all students must graduate with a bachelor's degree. Most of the acupuncture schools in the United States require a minimum of three years of full-time schooling to receive a master's degree in acupuncture. However, now, many acupuncture schools extend this to four years and offer doctor of acupuncture degrees. After they finish their study, they must take the national license exam (National Certification Commission for Acupuncture and Oriental Medicine [NCCAOM]) everywhere but California, which has its own acupuncture exam, and New Jersey, which requires an oral exam. Please visit the NCCAOM website for details.
2. Many acupuncturists graduated from foreign acupuncturist schools come to the United States. In spite of their different education, their schools must be accredited by the Accreditation Commission for Acupuncture and Oriental Medicine (ACAOM) (http://www.acaom.org), and all the acupuncturists must pass the exam of NCCAOM to receive their license from state governments in the United States.

Please check your acupuncturist's background by visiting your state's licensing agency. You may also call the acupuncturist's office to get further information regarding their training and see if they accept your insurance.

Most states require that non-physician acupuncturists pass an examination conducted by the NCCAOM: http://www.nccaom.org/.

MY PERSONAL ADVICE

1. The most important step is to check the background of the acupuncturist you wish to visit.

2. Ask for references. Good acupuncturists will always be happy to provide references.
3. Trust your instincts. If you do not feel good, do not go.

POSSIBLE REACTIONS TO ACUPUNCTURE

1. Sometimes you may feel faint and lightheaded after finishing an acupuncture treatment. It is a normal reaction—you might be too relaxed after the treatment and your blood pressure might be reduced. Do not worry; it is a good response to the treatment. Just wait a few minutes and then you will be OK to leave.
2. It sometimes happens that needles stick in the muscle because the muscle fibers get twisted around the needle. This is just a reflex, and your acupuncturist will gently remove the needle.
3. If the pain seems worse after the first treatment, this is a good sign. It means the energy flow is trying to heal the injury, and your body is adjusting your own balance to heal the problem.

6

Current Theories of Acupuncture in China

Acupuncture has been studied in China for thousands of years. Since 1949, the Chinese government has spent large amounts of money and organized many resources to study the meridians. The following theoretical phenomena were developed from their research.

MAIN HYPOTHESES OF THE MECHANISMS OF MERIDIANS

1. The meridians are related to the peripheral nerves. One group of scientists believes that the needles inserted into the acupuncture points will stimulate the nerve-sensation receptors, leading to an impulse transmitted to the central nervous system and causing a reaction in the internal organs.
2. The meridians are connected to nerve-ganglion distribution. Scientists think the meridians are correlated with the ganglion nerve, such as the cervical, thoracic, and lumbar ganglion nerve distribution.
3. The meridians are related to the central nervous system. Some scientists state that the meridians are not only transmitted through the body's surface but are also implanted in the central nervous system. As an example, amputees feel a pain in their missing leg, known as phantom pain. Even though their leg is gone, they still feel the pain, and this is because the meridians are implanted in the central nervous system.
4. The meridians are associated with the autonomic nervous system. This nervous system controls the heartbeat, sweating, and blood pressure. Some people who are undergoing acupuncture treatment may experience a faster or slower heartbeat, sweating,

or lower blood pressure, all of which indicate that the meridians might be associated with the autonomic nervous system.

5. The meridians are coupled with nerve-hormone systems. Acupuncture treatment might produce two types of reaction: a fast reaction from the nervous system and a slow reaction from the hormone system. This may explain why acupuncture can adjust endorphins and other brain peptides to increase or decrease in the brain.

6. The meridians are linked with the blood-lymph vessel system. A doctor injected a radioactive isotope into a fresh cadaver and then checked the isotope pathway. This experiment found that the isotope was indeed transmitted through the vein-lymph vessels, which would appear to prove that the meridians might also be linked with the blood-lymph vessel system.

7. The meridians are interconnected with the muscle-tendon-connective tissue. Many studies showed evidence that the meridian pathways may also follow a certain muscle-tendon-connective tissue structure.

ADDITIONAL HYPOTHESES OF THE MECHANISMS OF MERIDIANS

Meridian-Internal Organs-Cortical Hypotheses

In 1959, Dr. Xijun Zhang believed that the meridian distributions were connected to internal organs, such as liver, heart, and spleen, which were also connected to cortical-endocrine system. For example, Nei Guan (P6) was well known to slow down the heart rate by reducing the secretion of adrenocortical hormone.

The Third Balance System

Dr. Shaowei Meng thought there were four balance systems in the human body (see Table 6.1).

Double Reflection Circuit

Dr. Tong Wang indicated that by insertion of needles into the acupuncture points, there were two circuits excited; the long circuit was the central nervous system and the short reflection was through nerve ends/receptors due to activation of local enzyme and other chemicals.

Table 6.1

Balance Systems	Classification	Velocity	Function
1	Somatic nervous system	100 m/s	Fast posture balance
2	Autonomic nervous system	1 m/s	Internal organ balance
3	Meridian system	0.1 m/s	Body surface—organ balance
4	Endocrine system	Minutes	Whole-body slow balance

Network System of Meridian-Cell Gap

Dr. Yubao Ma thought that meridian was an independent regulating system. Meridian actually was a network system of meridian-cell gap through bioelectrophysiological energy.

New Autonomic System between Internal Organs and Body Surface

Dr. Puzhong Ji believed that there was a new networking system between internal organs and body surface. Meridians were the connecting system of both the internal organs and the body's surface.[1]

PART TWO

Theories of Traditional Chinese Medicine

7

The Theory of Yin and Yang

THE RELATIONSHIP OF YIN AND YANG TO NATURE

The theory of yin and yang is an observation and interpretation of the Chinese people to nature.

In 221 BC, the concept of yin and yang first appeared in *The Book of Changes*. "Yin and yang reflect all the forms and characteristics existing in the universe." Yin and yang are concepts of philosophy. Every object in the universe consists of the negative and the positive, and yin and yang represent the dynamic balance of opposites. Yin and yang are distinctively Chinese in terms of the perception of profound fundamental principles and as expressions of a unique way of viewing the world and the universe (see Figure 7.1).

Water and fire are used to symbolize the basic properties of yin and yang. Yang is life and growth; yin is death and storage. Yang is the body's surface, yin is the body's interior, and this is the same for every internal organ.

There are four relationships between yin and yang, and they are interconnected, with each one influencing the other and each being the cause or effect of the others. The four are inter-opposing, inter-depending, inter-consuming/supporting, and inter-transforming.

The following are some of the better-known examples of yin and yang that show their characteristics and their relationship to each other (see Table 7.1).

Yin and Yang Are Opposites

They are either on the opposite ends of a cycle, like the seasons of the year, or opposites on a continuum of energy or matter. This opposition is relative and can be spoken of only in relationships. They are in a

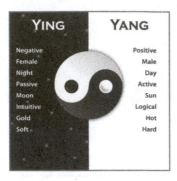

Figure 7.1

dynamic balance of many opposing forces. For example, night after midnight is yin relative to morning, but yang is relative to the time before midnight. Yin and yang are never static but are in a constantly changing balance.

The Infinite Division of Yin and Yang

Anything in this world can be divided into yin and yang, and they are in a constant state of change and can be divided indefinitely. In the body, the top half is yang and the bottom half is yin; the back is yang, and the front is yin; the left side is yang, and the right side is yin.

Yin and Yang Are Interdependent and Cannot Exist without Each Other

Nothing is totally yin or totally yang. Yin does not exist without yang and vice versa. For example, if there is no daytime, there will be no nighttime; if there is no concept of dark, there will be no light because they are mutually reliant on each other.

Yin and Yang Are in a State of Continuous Support

Relative levels of yin and yang are continuously changing. Normally, this is a harmonious change, but when yin or yang are out of balance, they affect each other, and too much of one can eventually weaken (consume) the other. For example, follow the sunrise in the morning and yin will gradually decrease. At noontime, yang will be in its strongest and most powerful stage; in the afternoon, however, yang will gradually decrease and yin will start to rise, and by night yang is almost gone and the

Table 7.1

Yin	Night	Moist	Cold	Water	Moon	Dark	Earth
Yang	Day	Dry	Warm	Fire	Sun	Bright	Sky

Yin	Rest	West	Right	Death	Small	Downward
Yang	Activities	East	Left	Birth	Large	Upward

predominant force is yin. That is true until midnight, when yang gradually starts to increase as yin gradually decreases; by morning, yang is rising again, demonstrating why yin and yang are mutually consuming and supporting.

Four Possible States of Imbalance

Excess of yin
Excess of yang
Deficiency of yin
Deficiency of yang

Mutually Dependent Aspects of Yin and Yang

Yin can change into yang and vice versa, but it is not a random event, happening only when the time is right. For example, spring comes only when winter is finished. Relatively, yin is down and yang is elevating. Yin and yang are two aspects of one mutually dependent phenomenon.

APPLYING THE YIN AND YANG THEORY TO TRADITIONAL CHINESE MEDICINE (TCM)

The Body's Structure

Relative to the structure of the human body, there are three aspects of yin and yang.

- *The location on the body.* As stated, the upper body is yang, and the lower body is yin; the external body is yang, and the interior body

Table 7.2

Yin	Chest	Body	Organs	Below waist	Anterior extremities	Body fluid	Solid organs
Yang	Back	Head	Skin, muscle	Above waist	Posterior extremities	Qi	Hollow organs

Yin	Heart	Lung	Liver	Spleen	Kidney	Pericardium
Yang	Small intestine	Large intestine	Gallbladder	Stomach	Bladder	San Jiao

is yin. The aspects of the four extremities toward the body's mid-line are yin, and the aspects of the four extremities away from the body's midline are yang.

- *The internal organ systems.* TCM physicians treat their patients using the yin-yang principle. The gallbladder, large intestine, small intestine, stomach, urinary bladder, and other organs with active movement are yang organs, known as the fu organs. The heart, kidney, liver, lung, and spleen and other organs with unper-ceptively active movement are yin organs, known as the Zang organs. Treatment for active yang organs is mainly to keep these organs moving. Treatment for the less-active yin organs consists mainly of acupuncture and Chinese herbs. This is to keep the vital energy of these inactive organs smooth.
- *The acupuncture meridian system.* Meridians are yin and yang. The yin organs are paired with the yin meridians, and the yang organs are paired with the yang meridians.

The Body's Physiological Function

All the functional activities of each of the organs are yang, but their activi-ties are also related to yin because yin substances are the various nutri-ents nourishing each of the organs. Yin supports the organ activities of the yang, and yang depends on yin nutrients to support them.

The Body's Pathological Changes

TCM applies the theory of yin and yang to pathological changes in the human body. The kidney, for example, is both yang and yin. If it has a yang deficiency, that will make the body feel cold and have lowered en-ergy, poor digestion, and stasis (a stoppage of the normal flow of a body substance); if it has a yin deficiency, the body will feel hot and thirsty; the person will sleep poorly and have low energy as well. Since yin and yang need to keep balanced in the body's organs, where there is any deficiency or excess, varying problems will arise in each organ (see Table 7.3).

Diagnosis and Treatment

When there is an imbalance of yin and yang in the organs causing differ-ent kinds of pathological changes, TCM can make a diagnosis based on these pathological changes. If someone reports having a stomachache, the practitioner first ascertains whether it is caused by a yang or yin excess or deficiency. A yang excess would be the case if the stomach has too much

Table 7.3

Yin	Yang
Inactive	Active
Deficiency	Excess
Sluggish activities	Hyperactivity
Chronic/gradual onset illness	Acute/rapid onset of illness
Slow development	Rapid changes
Quiet, lethargy, sleepiness	Restlessness, insomnia
Wants to be covered in the bed	Throws off comforter in bed
Sleep with curled position	Sleep with stretched-out position
Cold limbs and body	Hot limbs and body
Pale face	Red face
Weak voice, silent	Loud voice, talkative
Shallow, weak breathing	Coarse breathing
No thirst/wants warm drinks	Thirst prefer for cold drinks
Copious, clear urine	Scanty, yellow or dark urine
Loose stools (fluids not transformed)	Constipation (fluid evaporated by heat)
Clear, copious secretions	Thick, sticky white/yellow secretions
Excessive moisture	Excessive dryness (throat, skin, eyes, etc.)
Degenerative disease	Inflammatory disease
Pale tongue, white coat	Red tongue, yellow coat
Slow and weak pulse	Rapid and strong pulse

fire, and the person has a very strong appetite, a bad taste or smell in the mouth, some ulceration, or a toothache. If there is a yang deficiency, the person will also have a mild stomachache and will want to use warmth for it (e.g., drinking hot water).

Treatments for each case are completely different because the clinical diagnoses are different. If there is a yang excess in the stomach, the best treatment is to use Chinese herbs and acupuncture to purge the fire and the excess yang. When there is a yang deficiency in the stomach, herbs and acupuncture will also be used to improve the stomach yang. Again, with a yin excess, acupuncture points and Chinese herbs to intensify yang will be used to keep the yin-yang balance. The same applies if there is a yin deficiency—acupuncture points and Chinese herbs will be used to intensify yin. The herbs and acupuncture points selected will vary for each of these conditions and are a good demonstration of how diagnosis and treatment using the yin and yang theory can improve the stomach yang.

8

The Theory of Five Elements

The five elements theory is based on observation of the natural cycles and interrelationships in both the environment and the human body. The foundation of the theory rests on five categories in the natural world: wood, fire, earth, metal, and water (see Figure 8.1).

Everything in the universe corresponds to a variety of phenomena. The most common correspondences are listed in Table 8.1.

FIVE ELEMENTS CYCLES, RELATIONSHIPS, AND INTERACTIONS

Within the five elements theory, there are four main relationships or ways in which the elements interact.

1. *The generating (sheng, mother–child) cycle.* Each element, serving as a mother, promotes the growth and development of the other (child) element (see Figure 8.2).

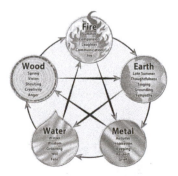

Figure 8.1

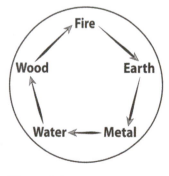

Figure 8.2

Table 8.1

	Fire	Earth	Metal	Water	Wood
Seasons	Summer	Late Summer	Autumn	Winter	Spring
Environment	Heat	Dampness	Dryness	Cold	Wind
Developmental Stages	Growth	Transformation	Harvest	Storage	Birth
Direction	South	Center	West	North	East
Yang Organs	Small intestine, San Jiao	Stomach	Large intestine	Urinary bladder	Gallbladder
Yin Organs	Heart	Spleen	Lung	Kidney	Liver
Sense Organs	Tongue	Mouth	Nose	Ears	Eyes
Tissues	Vessels	Muscles	Skin	Bone	Tendons
Tastes	Bitter	Sweet	Pungent	Salty	Sour
Colors	Red	Yellow	White	Blue/black	Green
Sounds	Laughing	Singing	Crying	Groaning	Shouting
Emotions	Joy	Worry/ pensiveness	Grief/ sadness	Fear	Anger

Based on Figure 8.2:

- Wood provides the generative force for fire;
- Fire enriches the earth;
- Earth contains metal;
- Metal produces water;
- Water nourishes wood;
- And so it goes.

From a clinical point of view, liver controls emotion, if the liver (wood) is strong, then the heart (fire) will start to burn. The burned fire (heart) will increase the nutrition of earth (spleen), the spleen (earth) will also enrich the lung (metal), the lung will produce water (kidney), and then the water will give birth to the wood (liver). Traditional Chinese medicine (TCM) tries to use the five elements theory to explain the relationship among the internal organs and their flow of mutual dependence.

2. *The controlling cycle* (ke, grandparent–grandchild). There is a check-and-balance system among all the elements. Earth, for example, provides a control for water and is controlled by wood. An example of this relationship within the body is in cases of anxiety (fire), which is related to liver qi stagnation (wood) where, over time, you begin to see more kidney-(water) related signs as the water element attempts to control the overactive fire (see Figure 8.3).
3. The overacting cycle (cheng). This is an imbalance within the controlling cycle where the grandmother element provides too much control over the grandchild and weakens the element. Within nature you may see water putting out fire, earth soaking up water, and so on (see Figure 8.3).

   A clinical example of this relationship would be liver (wood) overacting on the spleen (earth). In this case, you have an overactive wood element over controlling earth, leading to disruptions in the digestive system.
4. *The counteracting cycle* (wu) is also an imbalance within the controlling cycle where the grandchild insults or returns the controlling force generated by the grandmother. Using examples from nature you can see fire burning up water, and water washing away earth, and so on (see Figure 8.4).

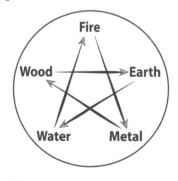

Figure 8.3

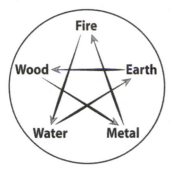

Figure 8.4

Clinically you may see that people have long-term psychological problems (fire), which eventually affect the kidneys (water) as seen in the development of more yin (water) deficiency signs.

THE FIVE ELEMENTS THEORY AND TRADITIONAL CHINESE MEDICINE

In TCM, the five elements theory is applied to the body's system of organs. For example, the liver is linked to wood, which grows and spreads out. This means that, just like wood, the functions of the liver will spread out and smoothly extend the liver's energy. Any interference in the liver's energy will make the liver unsteady, not a desirable outcome because, since the liver controls blood and emotion, it needs to be like wood, and it needs to always be growing.

In TCM, the heart is linked to fire, one of the five elements. The heart has little yin, so it functions as a pure yang machine, using the circulating blood system to pump yang energy upward, like fire, throughout the entire body.

9

The Theory of Zang-Fu Organs

THERE ARE FIVE ZANG ORGANS

Each of the five zang organs has its own individual function. All of them are coordinated in the harmony and balance of yin-yang, and they work together to make the body a uniform system. Because the zang organs deal predominately with blood, energy, and body fluid, they are called yin-zang, compared with yang-fu (discussed later in this chapter).

The Heart

The heart as a specific organ not only controls the blood and circulation but also dominates the mind, which is contrary to the belief of Western medicine.

- *The heart controls the blood* and the circulation, and demonstrates its function and capability on each person's face. Like an engine, it pumps blood through the blood vessels to the entire body. The stronger the engine, the more blood will be pumped to the body and face. The theory in traditional Chinese medicine (TCM) is that the heart dominates the blood vessels that manifests the heart's function on the face, so a TCM-trained physician can observe the heart's function by looking at a person's face. If it is flushed and ruddy, that means the person is in good health, but if it is pale, that means his or her heart function is not strong enough to nourish the entire body.
- *The heart hosts the mind.* The heart contains the function of mind and brain in TCM, which is similar to the Western concept, as, for example, with the often heard phrase "My heart is broken," which actually means "I am very sad."

- *The heart has an outlet through the tongue.* The tongue is the outer manifestation of the heart, and its color and shape indicate the condition of the heart. When the heart functions powerfully, it can push blood through the body, including to the tongue, and you will see a full red tongue. If, on the other hand, someone has anemia or loss of blood, you will see a pale tongue.

The Liver

- *The liver's main function is to be a warehouse for blood.* The liver stores the blood and regulates the blood volume by helping the heart regulate the blood circulation. If the heart has no power, the blood cannot be pumped through the body, thereby affecting all the body's normal functions. If the liver does not have enough blood, the person will look very pale, even though he or she may have a strong heart.
- *The liver regulates and manipulates the circulation and spreading of qi.* Qi is the energy of the body, and generally speaking, it supports the functioning of the entire body. Without control from the liver, qi will flow in a pathway that could cause complicated confusion and lead to abnormal functioning throughout the body. The liver has the following five sub-functions.

  - *Liver energy is related to emotions.* The liver, together with the brain, plays a role in emotional control. It usually sees when there is too little liver yin, which might cause, besides unsteady emotions, a bitter mouth, low energy, oversleep, or poor sleep. When liver yang is overwhelming, you will see a wide variety of symptoms and crazy behavior, such as anger, chest pains, dizziness, facial reddening, fitful sleep, high blood pressure, insomnia, irrational behavior, severe headaches, unpleasant dreams, vertigo, and similar. When liver qi is stagnant, that could manifest as depression, paranoia, and even weeping.
  - *The liver regulates the digestion.* The liver function is closely related to digestion. If, for example, somebody is too happy, too angry, or too focused on something, this person does not feel hungry and may not eat anything. This simple observation can lead to the conclusion that the liver's controlling emotion is closely connected with digestion—the excessive liver function (wood) will prohibit the stomach's ability (earth).
  - *The liver maintains muscles and tendons,* and a person's nails can show how it is functioning. This is because the liver, a storage

warehouse of blood, supplies all the needs of the joints, muscles, and tendons. If a deficiency or shortage of liver blood occurs, then these joints, muscles, and tendons will lack nourishment, and the low blood supply will limit their function, so it is possible to observe the liver blood deficiency by viewing the color of a person's nails—if there is not enough supply of liver blood, the nails will be pale.

- *The liver is related to supplying the entire body with blood.* In its main role as the storage facility for blood, the liver helps the heart pump blood out to entire body.
- *The liver has an outlet opening in the eye.* The liver stores blood, but a low blood supply can result in blurry vision, dry eyes, and night blindness. If there is too much liver fire, it can cause painful eyes, as well as facial redness and swelling.

The Spleen

The spleen mainly governs digestion and controls the blood. Its functions are as follows.

- *Transportation and transformation* are governed by the spleen. As soon as the stomach digests food and water, the spleen essentially transforms it into usable nutrition and energy (qi) and then transports these to other organs and the body's four extremities. In this function, the spleen plays an essential role in the production of qi, blood, and digestion.
- *The spleen can hold the blood inside the blood vessels.* Spleen qi is specifically responsible for keeping blood within the vessels. A weakness in this function can lead to chronic bleeding, including a tendency to bruise easily or experience breakthrough bleeding in the middle of the menstrual cycle.
- *The spleen governs the muscles and the four limbs.* The spleen is in charge of transforming food into qi and blood and transporting them throughout the body. It is, therefore, essential for maintaining joint flexibility, muscle mass, and strong limbs. A person with deficient spleen qi often experiences weakness and fatigue in the limbs.
- *The spleen opens into the mouth and manifests itself on the lips.* As the entrance to the digestive system, the mouth shows whether or not the spleen is functioning normally. If the spleen qi is normal, the spleen can transform and transport all the nourishments to the body, and as a result, the appetite is good, the lips are red and supple, and the sense of taste is sufficiently sensitive. If the spleen

is not normal, the appetite will be poor, the sense of taste will be impaired, possibly with a sticky sweetish sensation in the mouth, and the lips will be pale.

The Lung

The lung is the respiratory organ. It controls breathing through the inhalation of oxygen and the exhalation of carbon dioxide. Along with the spleen, the lung is also the source of postnatal qi, the vital life energy after a person is born.

- *The lung governs the qi (energy) of respiration and expels the qi throughout the whole body to nourish the organs.* The lung governs all the qi energy of the body and its organs because, comparable to an umbrella, it covers the entire body and all the organs. As such, it occupies the highest position of all the organs in the human body.
- *The lung transforms inhaled air into lung qi,* and for this reason, it plays an important role in the functional activities of the entire body. When the lung qi is strong, it can send this qi to the whole body and its internal organs to activate the body's function. Weak lung qi, on the other hand, will deprive the entire body and its internal organs of energy, leading to fatigue, low voice, shortness of breath, and the avoidance of external wind.
- *The lung also dominates the body's descending fluids and regulates the water passages.* All the fluid in the body will follow along the descending pathway of lung qi and spread out to the entire body. Since the lung is at the top of the body, its qi descends to circulate the entire body's qi and fluid. When this descending action of the lungs is interrupted and the normal flow of qi is blocked, coughing, shortness of breath, and other respiratory-tract illnesses may occur. Also, fluids may accumulate in the upper body, resulting in edema, difficulty in urination, and severe water retention in all four extremities and the abdomen.
- *The lung supports skin and hair.* This concept is based on the observation that human beings will cough and get cold if exposed to cold air for a long time. There must be some connection between the skin and lung, as observed. TCM believes the coldness attacks the lung, causes coughing, and makes people get colds through the hair holes. Body hair and pores are considered an integral part of the lungs' defensive system. They act as the boundary between the outer environment and the interior body, protecting it from an attack by the external environment. The qi that flows just under the skin is called *wei qi* and functions as the body's

immune system. When the wei qi is strong, the body is able to defend itself from external pathogens.

- *The nose is an opening for the lung.* It controls the voice and the respiratory and olfactory functions (breathing, smelling, and the voice) that depend on lung qi. When lung qi is healthy, the sense of smell is acute, the nasal passages remain open, and the voice is strong. When lung qi is dysfunctional, the person may experience symptoms of nasal congestion, excessive mucus, an impaired sense of smell, and a weak or hoarse voice.

The Kidneys

The kidneys are the energy house of the body, and they have the following functions.

- *Storage of essence (jing) and playing an important role in development and reproduction.* The kidneys store jing, or essence, a subtle substance that underlies all organic life processes. There are two types of essences (jing).

  1. Prenatal essence: Derived from the genetic materials of parents at birth, this unalterable prenatal essence is a very important gift from parents. It provides an origin of life and determines the physical body and mental character of a person; for example, tall, thin parents usually have tall, thin children, and mentally and physically healthy parents most likely have healthy children.
  2. Postnatal essence: this essence, on the other hand, is within a person's control and is changeable. It is possible for a person who has a weak prenatal essence to lead a vital, healthy life through the maintenance of a strong postnatal essence. A healthy diet and lifestyle, fully developed, normal, mental capacity, along with physical exercise, are the means to achieving strong postnatal essence. In fact, a person with a weak constitution and a healthy lifestyle is better off than a person with a strong constitution and an unhealthy lifestyle.

Working together, the prenatal and postnatal essences contribute to the reproductive essence. The kidneys store this reproductive essence and maintain the reproductive life.

- *The kidneys control the reception of qi from other organs.* Because the kidneys store the essence, their qi can control and support other qi transportation from the liver, lung, spleen, and stomach. Only when the kidney qi is strong and there is enough of the kidney's essence will the passage of qi in the lung be active and the stomach and spleen qi functional.

- *The kidney is very important in water metabolism.* When the kidney qi is out of balance, many people often have edema, difficulty voiding, prolonged urination, or water retention. The balance of yin and yang in the kidneys determines the efficiency of water metabolism in the body.
- *The kidneys can produce bone marrow,* and as a result, they can control bone density and are connected to the brain. Marrow, including both bone marrow and brain tissue, is derived directly from essence, and this is the source of the substance that makes up the brain. Deficiencies in essence or marrow can appear in cases of osteoporosis, headaches, and mental retardation.
- *The kidney qi supports hearing.* Older people can develop impaired hearing or have a ringing in the ears (tinnitus), due to a depletion of their kidney qi (essence) over time. Clinically, hearing difficulties can often be treated by nourishing the kidneys with Chinese herbs or acupuncture.
- *A kidney deficiency can show itself in the hair.* The hair can turn gray and even white when people become older because the hair relies on nourishment by the kidney essence to grow.

The Pericardium

The pericardium is a membrane shielding the heart. It protects the heart from pathological qi.

THERE ARE SIX FU ORGANS

Except for San Jiao, the fu organs are very similar to all the functions of the same-name organs in Western medicine.

The Gallbladder

The major function of the gallbladder is the storage and excretion of bile. It is also responsible for judgment and thoughts, such as dreams or fears.

The Stomach

Grinding and digestion is the major function of the stomach.

The Small Intestine

Absorbing the essence of the food and separating it from unwanted nutrition are the functions of the small intestine.

The Large Intestine

The large intestine is responsible for transportation. It absorbs water and transports the wastes out the body.

The Urinary Bladder

The responsibility of the urinary bladder is to store fluid and excrete urine.

San Jiao

San Jiao is not a clearly understood organ. Its role is to host and separate the functions of the organs in the upper, middle, and lower three parts of the body, along the chest and abdominal cavities.

10

The Theory of Meridians

Meridians are channels that transfer blood and energy throughout the body, and they are connected with the surface and all the internal organs of the body. Clinically, there are 14 major meridians, 12 of them symmetrically distributed on both sides of the body, plus several minor meridians, which are used to connect the body to every cell and nerve. The meridians are used to guide clinical diagnoses and the treatment of many diseases.

THE SIX PAIRS OF MERIDIANS

- Lung and large intestine meridians
- Stomach and spleen meridians
- Heart and small intestine meridians
- Urinary bladder and kidney meridians
- Pericardium and San Jiao meridians
- Gallbladder and liver meridians

THE DU AND REN MERIDIANS

The Du meridian travels mainly along the midline of the back, and the Ren meridian travels along the midline of the chest and abdomen.

THE MAIN FUNCTION OF THE MERIDIANS

The meridians connect all the internal organs with the body's surface, including all the joints, muscles, nerves, and skin, which form the body into one highly organized whole.

- They regulate yin and yang, and transport qi (energy) and blood through their channels.
- They have strong defensive connections that resist and prevent the invasion of pathogens. They also transport blood and qi to attack the invasive pathogens.
- In addition, they transport the sensation and the energy of the acupuncture needle and regulate the deficiency or excess of conditions in the body. The meridian theory guides the practitioner in the following ways.
- *Observation* Because the meridians connect the internal organs, an illness in any of them is observed on the face and skin. For example, the heart's color is red, the lung's is white, the liver's is dark blue, the spleen's is yellow, and the kidney's is black. Any excessive, disproportionate color on the face or body can indicate disease in a particular internal organ.
- *Palpation* By palpating (feeling) the pulse on the lateral wrist, the energy and blood of an internal organ can be detected. If, for example, the pulse is too rapid, this can indicate heat in the internal organ, or that the emotions are too strong.
- *Points selection* After making a clear diagnosis based on the theory of traditional Chinese medicine, the acupuncturist can choose acupuncture points from the different meridians. Different combinations of the points and meridians can treat different diseases.

Acupuncture Points

Acupuncture points are the locations along each of the specific meridians used for the insertion of needles. There are about 400 frequently used points.

HOW THE MERIDIANS ARE LABELED

There are about 400 commonly used acupuncture points along the 14 meridians. With about a 3,000-year history, all the points are named in Chinese; each point has a specific function and meaning, and a role related to its internal organ and meridian. There are also around 50 points not located within the standard meridians, which are called extraordinary points. Because of the complexity and difficulty of these Chinese names, the WHO has tried to standardize them with numbers (see Table 10.1).

Table 10.1 The Naming Regulations and Abbreviations of Meridian and Acupuncture Points

No	Meridian Name	Abbrev	Acu point Starts	Acu Point Ends	No	Meridian Name	Abbrev	Acu point Starts	Acu Point Ends
1	Lung	Lu	Lu 1	Lu 11	2	Large intestine	LI	LI 1	LI 20
3	Stomach	St	St 1	St 45	4	Spleen	Sp	Sp 1	Sp 21
5	Heart	Ht	Ht 1	Ht 9	6	Small intestine	SI	SI 1	SI 19
7	Urinary Bladder	UB	UB 1	UB 67	8	Kidney	Ki	Ki 1	Ki 27
9	Pericardium	Pc	Pc 1	Pc 9	10	San Jiao	SJ	SJ 1	SJ 23
11	Gallbladder	Gb	Gb 1	Gb 44	12	Liver	Li	Li 1	Li 14
13	Du	Du	Du 1	Du 28	14	Ren	Ren	Ren 1	Ren 24

PATHWAYS OF THE TWELVE MAIN MERIDIANS

The 12 main meridians are distributed throughout the body. Via the internal organs and surface of the body, they are connected with each other in an endless cycle to nourish and adjust the energy of the body.

To begin with the meridian lung, it is connected to the large intestine, then the stomach, the spleen, the heart, the small intestine, the urinary bladder, the kidney, the pericardium, the San Jiao, the gallbladder, the liver, and finally back to the lung again.

PART THREE

Case Histories

11

Cervical Dystonia

Matthew, an 18-year-old young man, was brought to see me by his mother because, about six years before, when he woke up one morning, he suddenly realized that his neck had turned to the left and was accompanied by a sudden involuntary jerk. From that time forward, his neck continued to jerk suddenly and turn to the left. The involuntary jerks were very frequent, he said, occurring two or three times every five to ten minutes, and they got worse when he was tired or under stress. If he had gotten a good night's sleep, however, and was energetic or focused on something, such as the sports he likes, he said he never had the sudden, involuntary neck movement. It occurred only when he sat without doing anything. His neck muscle was always very tight, he said, and sometimes painful. Matthew went to many doctors and tried many different medications with no improvement. Finally, he came to me for evaluation and treatment (see Figure 11.1).

I performed a physical examination that showed exaggerated muscle growth on the left side of his neck, especially the main neck muscle, the sternocleidomastoid, which felt like big rope. I also felt other muscles that had increased in bulk, for example, the levator scapular at the back of the neck and the splenius capitis. During the entire physical examination, Matthew had no jerks or involuntary contractions on the left side of his neck.

What Matthew was experiencing is called cervical dystonia, the most common form of a localized movement disorder called focal dystonia.

SYMPTOMS, CAUSES, AND DIAGNOSIS

Dystonia is a chronic, often painful, neurological disorder characterized by loss of control over one or more parts of the body where muscle

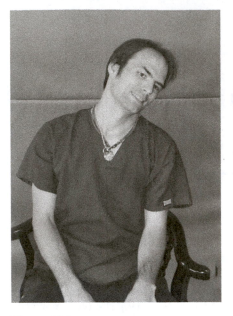

Figure 11.1

contractions cause twisting or abnormal postures that can affect a single muscle or a group of muscles, such as those in arms, neck, legs, or the entire body.[1]

Cervical dystonia is diagnosed when there are twisting muscle contractions, repetitive movements, and spasmodic squeezing in the neck. The movement is involuntary and can sometimes be very painful, resulting in abnormal posture of the head and the neck area. The sustained, involuntary muscle contraction can cause severe, chronic neck pain that can hinder movement. It can occur in all ages, and women are twice as likely to be affected as men. People with dystonia usually have normal intelligence and no associated psychiatric disorders. Although cervical dystonia affects approximately 125,000 people in the United States alone, the cause of cervical dystonia is unknown and few people are aware of the condition.

Types of Cervical Dystonia

There are two types of cervical dystonia.

Primary cervical dystonia. This type is not related to any identifiable acquired disorders affecting the brain or spinal cord, such as an infection, stroke, trauma, or tumor. In primary cervical dystonia, some families were found to have an abnormal gene, *dystonia DYT1*, which could mean the condition is inherited. But not everyone carrying the *DYT1* gene will develop cervical dystonia, so it is therefore more likely that other genes or environmental factors play a role in the development of this type of cervical dystonia.

Secondary cervical dystonia. There is an obvious reason or cause that leads to the cervical dystonia, such as a stroke, a tumor, an infection in the brain or spinal cord, a traumatic brain injury, exposure to toxins, or a birth injury. There can be period of months between the underlying cause and the onset of cervical dystonia.

Tests and Diagnosis

The standard procedure is to rule out the secondary cervical dystonia. The following tests may be used to screen for cervical dystonia.

- Screening for toxins and infections by checking the blood or urine.
- Screening for tumors. An MRI will identify and visualize any tumors of the brain or spinal cord.
- Genetic testing can be used to identify if *DYT1* is present, and this will help with the diagnosis of primary cervical dystonia.
- Electromyography. This test measures the electrical activity of muscles. It can help in diagnosing muscle and nerve disorders and confirming the diagnosis.

TREATMENTS FOR CERVICAL DYSTONIA IN WESTERN MEDICINE

Noninvasive Treatments

Medications and physical therapy are the principal noninvasive methods of treatment for this condition.

Medications

Many different medications are tried in the treatment of cervical dystonia, but most of them do not work. For reference, they are as follows.

- Drugs that decrease the level of acetylcholine, such as Cogentin and Kemadrin, have worked for a few people, but they have undesirable sedating side effects.
- Drugs that regulate the neurotransmitter GABA, such as Valium, Ativan, or Klonopin.
- Drugs that either increase or decrease your dopamine level, such as Sinemet or Laridopa.
- Anticonvulsants, such as carbamazepine.

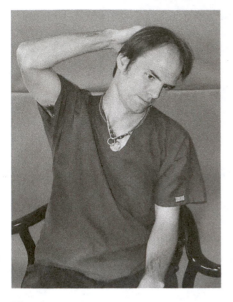

Figure 11.2

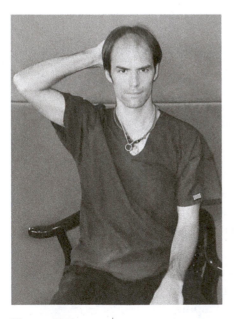

Figure 11.3

Physical Therapy

Physical therapy can be beneficial to help reduce stress, which cervical dystonia often exacerbates in tension-filled moments. Therapies can include deep breathing, meditation, or shifting your attention to a pleasant event to help resolve symptoms during an attack.

Another therapy is for the therapist to help you learn any sensory tricks, or *geste antagoniste* (moving an arm to the face or head). These sensory tricks can include having you apply hand pressure on your face, or press your head back into a chair or pillow to alleviate the dystonic posture during the episode. Though not fully understood, this is a well-known therapy that can help alleviate the abnormal posture of anyone with cervical dystonia (see Figures 11.2 and 11.3).

Invasive Treatments

Botox Injections, Surgery, and Deep Brain Stimulation

Botox can usually stop muscle spasms by blocking acetylcholine, and it usually relieves the symptoms in about three months.[2] However, a Botox injection must be done by very experienced hands. If it is used for more than a one-year period, its effects will gradually decrease because of auto-antibodies produced against the Botox.

In some severe cases, surgery might be a choice, but this is considered the treatment of last resort. The surgery, selective denervation, involves cutting the nerves supplying the muscles and, in some cases, cutting the muscles themselves.[3]

Another tactic is called deep brain stimulation, which involves implanting an electrode in the brain connected to a device in the chest that can be stimulated to generate an electrical pulse. These electrodes will temporarily disable nerve activities by damaging small areas of the brain.

TREATMENTS FOR CERVICAL DYSTONIA IN TRADITIONAL CHINESE MEDICINE

Chinese medicine thinks cervical dystonia is caused by excessive liver wind because liver functions control the movement of all the tendons, muscles, and joints of human body. If liver wind is excessive, the tendons, muscles, and joints will be overstimulated, and the muscle will constantly be activated.

Acupuncture

The principal treatment in acupuncture will be to decrease the activities of the tendons, muscles, and joints. The acupuncture points will be selected mainly from the meridians of the liver and Du, such as Du20 Bai Hui, GB20 Feng Chi, and Liv3 Tai Chong. However, anyone with this condition usually has an abnormal head movement, and the head belongs to the Du meridian that supplies the entire brain. If the Du meridian has been attacked by excessive liver wind, the entire head will continue to move; therefore, the acupuncturist will pick up the points of Du14 Da Zhui and Du19 Hou Ding from the Du meridian. These points will adjust and regulate the Du meridian, activate the tendon function, and balance the input and output of the Du meridian.

In addition, the acupuncturist will pick up UB 15 Xin Shu, a direct outlet from the heart, UB 23 Shen Shu, a connecting point from the kidney, Ht 7 Sheng Men, and Ki 3 Tai Xi. All these points will circulate in the heart and kidney and make the kidney and heart fire go down, therefore keeping the yin and yang in a harmonious situation. Some local points, such as SI 16 Tian Chuang, SI 17 Tian Rong, LI 17 Tian Ding, and LI 18 Fu Tu, are selected to calm the local area. The combination of local and distal points will usually greatly decrease the symptoms of cervical dystonia (see Table 11.1 and Figures 11.4 to 11.8).

Table 11.1

	Points	Meridian/ Number	Location	Conditions Helped
1	Bai Hui	Du 20	On the midline of the head, across the line of the two ear tips	Headaches, vertigo, tinnitus, nasal obstruction, apoplexy-induced aphasia, coma, mental disorders, prolapse of the rectum and the uterus
2	Feng Chi	Gallbladder point 20	In the depression between the upper portion of m. sternocleidomastoideus and m. trapezius, on the same level with Feng Fu (Du 16)	Headaches, vertigo, insomnia, pain and stiffness of the neck, blurred vision, glaucoma, red and painful eyes, tinnitus, convulsions, epilepsy, infantile convulsions, fever diseases, common cold, nasal obstruction, nose cold
3	Tai Chong	Liv 3	On the dorsum of the foot, in the depression distal to the junction for the 1st and 2nd metatarsal bones	Headaches, dizziness, and vertigo, insomnia, congestion, swelling and pain in the eyes, depression, infantile convulsions, deviation of the mouth, uterine bleeding, hernia, bedwetting, retention of urine, epilepsy
4	Da Zhui	Du 14	Below the spinous process of the 7th cervical vertebra, approximately at the level of the shoulders	Neck pain and rigidity, malaria, febrile diseases, epilepsy, afternoon fever, cough, asthma, common cold, back stiffness
5	Hou Ding	Du 19	On the midline of the back of head	Headaches, vertigo, mania, epilepsy

(Continued)

58

Table 11.1 *(Continued)*

	Points	Meridian/ Number	Location	Conditions Helped
6	Xin Shu (heart)	UB 15	1.5 inches lateral to midspine, at the level of lower border of the spinous process of the 5th thoracic vertebra	Cardiac pain, panic, loss of memory, palpitation, cough, spitting of blood, nocturnal emissions, night sweating, mania, epilepsy
7	Shen Shu	UB 23	1.5 inches lateral to the anterior body midline, at the level of the lower border of the spinous process of the 2nd lumbar vertebra	Nocturnal emission, impotence, bedwetting, irregular menstruation, vaginal discharge, low back pain, weakness of the knee, blurring of vision, dizziness, tinnitus, deafness, edema, asthma, diarrhea
8	Shen Men	HT 7	At the ulnar end of the transverse crease of the wrist, in the depression on the radial side of the tendon of flexor carpi ulnaris	Cardiac pain, irritability, palpitation, hysteria, amnesia, insomnia, mania, epilepsy, dementia, feverish sensation in the palm
9	Tai Xi	Ki 3	In the depression between the medial malleolus and tendon calcaneus, at the level of the tip of the medial malleolus	Sore throat, toothache, deafness, tinnitus, dizziness, spitting blood, asthma, thirst, irregular menstruation, insomnia, nocturnal emissions, impotence, frequency of urination, low back pain
10	Tian Chuang	SI 16	In the side of the neck, in the posterior border of m. sternocleidomastoideus, above Fu Tu	Sore throat, sudden loss of voice, deafness, tinnitus, stiffness and pain of the neck

(Continued)

Table 11.1 (*Continued*)

	Points	Meridian/ Number	Location	Conditions Helped
11	Tian Rong	SI 17	Posterior to the angle of mandible, in the depression on the anterior border of m. sternocleido-mastoideus	Deafness, tinnitus, sore throat, swelling of the cheek, foreign body sensation in the throat, goiter
12	Tian Ding	LI 17	On the lateral side of the neck, 1 inch below neck-Fu Tu point, on the posterior border of m. sternocleidomas-toideus	Sudden loss of voice, sore throat, scrofula, goiter
13	Fu Tu	LI 18	On the lateral side of the neck, level with the tip of Adam's apple, between the sternal head and clavicular head of m. sterno-cleidomastoideus	Cough, asthma, sore throat, sudden loss of voice, goiter

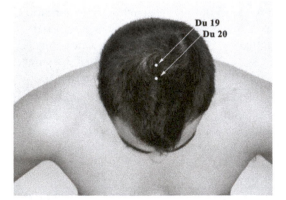

Figure 11.4

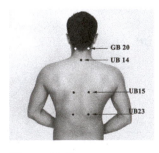

Figure 11.5

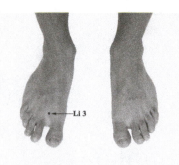

Figure 11.6

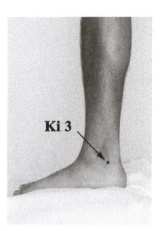

Figure 11.7

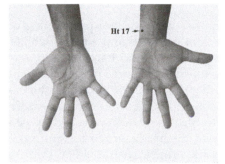

Figure 11.8

MATTHEW'S TREATMENT

Matthew was treated with the previously mentioned acupuncture points for about two months, three times a week, and after the last treatment, his neck contractions were greatly diminished. As of now, he basically has a mild neck jerk and mild contractions, and he can perform his daily studies very well.

TIPS FOR PEOPLE WITH CERVICAL DYSTONIA

- The earlier the treatment, the better the treatment results.
- Help yourself with massages and a heating pad.

TIPS FOR ACUPUNCTURE PRACTITIONERS

- Acupuncture cannot treat all types of cervical dystonia. The milder the disease, the better the treatment results.
- A heating pad plus a massage are very helpful after acupuncture treatment.

12

Occipital Neuralgia

Linda is a 45-year-old dental assistant who came to me complaining of severe headaches that started at the back of her head and went down her neck. The pain also radiated up to her scalp, around her ears, and was sometimes behind her right eye or into the temporal area on both sides of the head, as well as the top of her scalp. The pain was on and off, but it occurred every day—sometimes it was dull and sometimes sharp. Because of her profession, she very often had to turn her head to the right when dealing with her patients, and this caused the headaches to become more severe and interfered with her daily work, which frustrated her. Prior to visiting me, she had consulted several doctors for this condition and had been prescribed Naprosyn, Percocet, and Neurontin, but none of these alleviated her condition.

The headaches seemed to intensify when Linda was under stress, which happened frequently due to her job. If she had many patients waiting for her and felt under pressure, the headaches got worse.

When she consulted me for the problem, I examined her and discovered that when I pressed her scalp at the base of the skull (the suboccipital area), the pain radiated to the back, front, and side of her head, as well as to the right side of her eye. When I pressed harder on the suboccipital area, the pain was exacerbated. I could

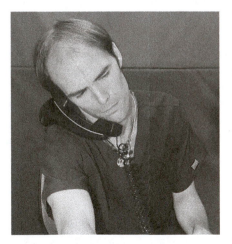

Figure 12.1 The tilted head position exacerbates the symptoms of headache.

feel her temporal arteries pulsating on both sides of her head, and I determined that Linda probably had an inflammation of the occipital nerves known as occipital neuralgia. And she exhibited the severe form of occipital neuralgia, most likely because her profession caused her to tilt her head in the same manner for a good part of her day. This caused the pinched occipital nerve, which sent the constant signal to the nerve network in her scalp, resulting in these headaches as well as the pain behind her right eye (see Figure 12.1).

SYMPTOMS, CAUSES, AND DIAGNOSIS

Occipital neuralgia is a cycle of pain spasms originating in the suboccipital area. There are two pairs of occipital nerves, the greater and lesser occipital nerves, and they originate in the area of the second and third vertebrae of the neck. They supply areas of the skin along the base of the skull and behind the ear, though they sometimes do not connect directly to the structures within the skull. However, they do interconnect with other nerves outside the skull and continue into the neural network. Eventually they can affect any given area throughout the scalp, mainly on the bilateral temporal area behind the ears, and can sometimes connect to the nerve branch on either side of both eyes.

Occipital neuralgia can occur continuously, often as the result of a pinched nerve, especially from arthritis, a muscle spasm, or as the result of a prior injury or surgery. Sometimes these conditions will pinch the occipital nerve root, causing a severe headache at the back of the head leading to muscle spasms.

In diagnosing occipital neuralgia, it is very important to assess posture to help to restore neutral alignment because very often such work as being a dental assistant who always turns to one side, or having a desk job sitting and answering phone call after phone call, or just typing at a computer all day, can cause repetitive strain where overused muscles get tight, and the end result is pain. The clinical diagnosis of this condition is based on the doctor's examination of the bilateral occipital nerve root with his or her fingers, which will induce or trigger the headache.

TREATMENTS FOR OCCIPITAL NEURALGIA
IN WESTERN MEDICINE

Noninvasive Treatments

Noninvasive treatments for this severely painful condition can include pain medications and physical therapy.

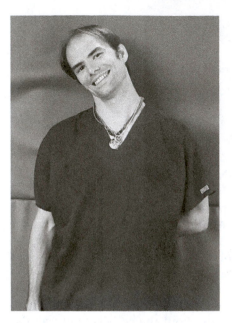

Figure 12.2   Bending your neck laterally and backward will help you stretch the opposite trapezius muscle.

Medications

Western medicines include anti-inflammatories or narcotics, such as Darvocet, Percocet, and Neurontin, or anti-epilepsy medication. Much of the time these medications do not work well, though occasionally they can reduce the occurrence and frequency of occipital neuralgia.

Physical Therapy

Some people respond to physical therapy and massages to decrease the spasms of the neck muscle and temporarily relieve this painful condition. Treatment can include instruction on how to stretch to loosen tight structures and then on how to strengthen weakened muscles to maintain proper alignment. This includes stretches to the upper trapezius and exercises for the middle trapezius, as shown in Figures 12.2 and 12.3. These movements, along with relaxation methods, will help combat the intensifying issues that often arise under stressful conditions.

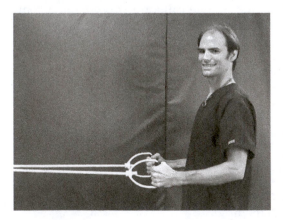

Figure 12.3

Invasive Treatments

Injections

The occipital nerve can sometimes be blocked by injecting 5 cc of 1 percent lidocaine to the nerve root, decreasing or relieving the pain, so the doctor can confirm the diagnosis and decide what medication would be most effective. Another treatment is a small injection of Botox.

Surgery

Sometimes surgery is required to cut the nerve or burn it with a radial wave probe. Though surgery may seem to be called for, many resist this type of treatment.

TREATMENTS FOR OCCIPITAL NEURALGIA IN TRADITIONAL CHINESE MEDICINE

Traditional Chinese medicine (TCM) thinks occipital neuralgia belongs in the category of side headache. The gallbladder meridians are distributed around the side of the head, so TCM believes that this side headache is caused by excessive heat in the gallbladder. The gallbladder meridian originates from the outside of the eye and continues up the temporal nerve area, then around it, down the occipital nerve area, and down through the trunk of the body to the outside of the leg. If there is excessive heat following this meridian, it will affect the balance of yin and yang, and if you experience stress, muscle spasms, or arthritis, the nerve and the gallbladder meridian will be affected. This will then cause the gallbladder to heat up, leading to excessive heat and creating poor balance of the yin and yang that will result in a severe headache. Meantime, there is the urinary bladder meridian that starts from the inside corner of the eye, continues to the middle, then the top, of the scalp and follows down the trunk and the back of the trunk into the back of the leg. Due to the connection between the gallbladder and urinary bladder meridians, heat in one will cause heat to rise in the other, and this will cause pain around the eye, the temporal area, and the scalp, making the ensuing headache severe and unbearable. The principal treatment for relieving this excessive heat in the meridians of gallbladder and urinary bladder is acupuncture.

Acupuncture

Usually acupuncture, with or without the addition of herbal supplements, can give good results to anyone with these types of headaches. Sometimes, however, it is best to combine acupuncture with a nerve block, utilizing 4 cc of 1 percent lidocaine plus 10 mg Kenalog, mixed together and injected into the origins of both sides of the occipital nerve. One month of this combined treatment should give 95 percent relief from the symptoms.

The main acupuncture points are Du 20 Bai Hui, GB 20 Feng Chi, GB1 Tong Zi Liao, GB 8 Shuai Gu, Extra point Tai Yang, GB 34 Yang Ling Quan, Hou Xi, Lie Que, Zhao Hai, and Liv 3 Tai Chong (see Table 12.1 and Figures 12.4 and 12.5).

Table 12.1

	Points	Meridian/ Number	Location	Conditions Helped
1	Bai Hui	Du 20	*See* Table 11.1/ Figure 11.4	*See* Table 11.1
2	Feng Chi	GB 20	*See* Table 11.1/ Figure 11.5	*See* Table 11.1
3	Tong Zi Liao	GB 1	0.5 inches lateral to the outer canthus, in the depression on the lateral side of the orbit	Headaches, redness and pain of the eyes, failing vision, tearing, deviation of the eye and mouth
4	Shuai Gu	GB 8	Superior to the apex of the auricle, 1.5 inches within the hairline	Migraine, vertigo, vomiting, infantile convulsions
5	Tai Yang	Extra point	In the depression about 1 inch posterior to the midpoint between the lateral end of the eyebrow and outer canthus	Headaches, eye diseases, deviation of the eyes and mouth
6	Yang Ling Quan	GB 34	In the depression anterior and inferior to the head of the fibula	Paralysis, weakness, numbness, and pain of the lower extremities, swelling and pain of the knee, beriberi, upper abdominal pain, bitter taste in the mouth, vomiting, jaundice, infantile convulsions
7	Hou Xi	SI 3	When a loose fist is made, the point is on the ulnar side, proximal to the 5th meta carpophalangeal joint, at the end of the trans	Pain and rigidity of the neck, tinnitus, deafness, sore throat, mania, malaria, acute lumbar sprain, night sweating, febrile diseases, contracture,

(Continued)

Table 12.1 (*Continued*)

Points	Meridian/ Number	Location	Conditions Helped
		verse crease and the junction of the red and white skin	and numbness of the fingers, pain in the shoulder and elbow
8 Lie Que	Lu 7	Superior to the styloid process of the radius, 1.5 inches above the transverse crease of the wrist	Headaches, migraine, neck rigidity, cough, asthma, sore throat, facial paralysis, toothache, pain, and weakness of the wrist
9 Zhao Hai	Kid 6	In the depression of the lower border of the medial malleolus, or 1 inch below the medial malleolus	Irregular menstruation, excessive vaginal discharge, prolapse of uterus, itching in the vulva, frequency of urination, retention of urine, constipation, epilepsy, insomnia, sore throat, asthma
10 Tai Chong	Li 3	*See* Table 11.1/ Figure 11.6, Figure 12.6.	*See* Table 11.1

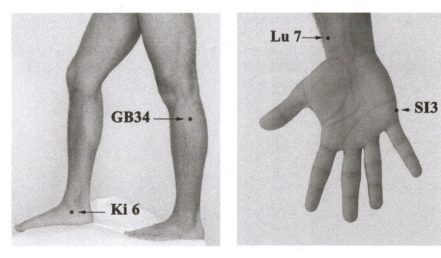

Figure 12.4

Figure 12.5

LINDA'S TREATMENT

Linda underwent my treatment three times a week for a month, which gave her immediate relief from her headaches. However, due to her strenuous work, the headaches returned later to plague her. Furthermore, she had an irregular period, and the hormonal changes connected with that triggered a severe headache as well, so I used a Chinese herb to treat her for these changes. The combination of acupuncture and herbal therapy seemed to be effective, and after about two months of treatment, Linda reported that her headaches were infrequent and very mild, and she was satisfied with her treatments.

TIPS FOR PEOPLE WITH OCCIPITAL NEURALGIA

- You should accurately describe the specific tender points on your head because different locations in the head belong to different meridians, and the treatment is different.
- Massage the Tai Yang and UB 20 Feng Chi points for 20 minutes, two to three times a day. This will greatly decrease your headache.

TIPS FOR ACUPUNCTURE PRACTITIONERS

- You should identify the location of the tender point, and treat the headache accordingly. The frontal headache belongs to the Yang Ming meridian, the temporal side headache belongs to the Shao Yang meridian, and the top of the scalp headache belongs to the Jue Ying meridian. You should choose the corresponding acupuncture points.
- Always use Du 20 Bai Hui for all different kinds of headaches. In my 20 years of practice, this has been my personal choice, and I have experienced much success with it.

13

Trigeminal Neuralgia

After Thomas, a 65-year-old man, had experienced a toothache on the right side of his mouth for a month, he finally consulted his dentist, who found two loose teeth on the right side at the back of his mouth. Thomas loves sweets, which may have caused the problem, but the pain was so severe that he was unable to sleep. The pain started when Thomas tried to brush his teeth, and it was so acute that he could not bear to touch his teeth or the right side of his face and jaw. Even currents of air triggered the pain. In addition to brushing his teeth, he had difficulty eating, talking, and shaving. The pain, unbearable at times, was stabbing, like electrical shocks, burning, and sometimes shooting. It attacked the right side of the jaw and face and lasted for hours. In order to avoid triggering an episode of pain, he intentionally tried not using the teeth on the right side of his mouth. Finally, the dentist decided to pull out his two lower teeth, at which point he felt immediate swelling on the right side of his face, and after a week, the pain became worse. The doctor prescribed narcotics to ease the pain, but when there was no improvement after the tooth extraction and Thomas could not touch the right side of his face, he decided to come to me.

Upon examining him, I discovered that although the pain did not extend to the right side of his eye, his right cheek and jaw were so tender that he described the pain as intolerable. Thomas felt it was incapacitating him to the extent that he was losing normal function; he had dropped 10 pounds, was experiencing fatigue, and was unable to sleep. My diagnosis was that Thomas had a severe case of trigeminal neuralgia affecting two of the three branches of the nerve, the V2 and V3.

SYMPTOMS, CAUSES, AND DIAGNOSIS

The trigeminal nerve carries sensation from the face to the brain. Many studies indicate that if this nerve is compressed by an overlying artery or vein in the brain, this compression injures the nerves protecting the myelin sheath, which causes erratic and hyperactive functioning of the nerve. This can lead to attacks of pain with the slightest stimulation of any area served by the nerve, and can hinder the nerve's ability to shut down pain signals when the stimulation ends. The trigeminal is the fifth cranial nerve, which registers sensory data, such as pressure and temperature, and measures pain originating from the face above the jaw line. The trigeminal nerve has three branches—one going to the eye, the second to the mouth, and the third to the jaw. I determined that Thomas could be affected by two branches of the trigeminal nerve.

This condition is usually found more in men (three men to every two women) and the causes of most trigeminal neuralgia cases are unknown. They typically occur in the sixth decade of life but may occur at any age, with symptoms from the secondary trigeminal nerve often showing up in younger people.

The most important factor in the diagnosis of trigeminal nerve neuralgia is the person's history. The pain can be brief, but it can also occur in multiple attacks and can be stabbing, shock like, or extremely severe. It is usually distributed along one or more branches of the trigeminal nerve and is usually in the upper or lower jaw on one side. This pain usually lasts from a few seconds to one to two minutes and will typically attack a few months a year.

TREATMENTS FOR TRIGEMINAL NEURALGIA IN WESTERN MEDICINE

Noninvasive Treatments

There are four main methods of treatment for this acutely painful condition; three of them are noninvasive; the fourth is surgery.

Medications

The ones most usually prescribed are anticonvulsants, including carbamazepine, phenytoin, or gabapentin. These are generally the most effective at relieving pain and can be used along with such muscle relaxants as baclofen. Some opioids, OxyContin or Duragesic in patch form, for example, can also be effective for decreasing pain in the jaw and face, as can low doses of antidepressants, such as amitriptyline.

Stereotactic Radiation Therapy

This procedure is done by a surgeon using a gamma knife or linear accelerator and is based on radiation therapy, such as Novalis CyberKnife, where the therapy penetrates the skin, targets the selective nerve root, and disrupts the transmissions of pain signals.

Physical Therapy

Physical therapy can be used to assess sleeping posture in order to improve the quality of sleep and allow you to wake up without pain. And giving an ice massage to muscles of the neck and jaw can help keep those areas relaxed.

Invasive Treatment

Surgery

Surgery might relieve pressure on the nerve through selective truncating of the nerve, which involves disrupting the pain signals to keep them from getting through to the brain, and is usually 90 percent successful if done by an experienced surgeon. The most specific instance of this is microvascular decompression, which involves open surgery to relieve the pressure of a blood vessel on the nerve.

TREATMENTS FOR TRIGEMINAL NEURALGIA IN TRADITIONAL CHINESE MEDICINE

Chinese medicine thinks that the stomach meridian goes around the eye, the jaw, and the teeth. Therefore, if there is blockage in the stomach meridian, the external wind and heat will be mixed together, and the wind flame will spread out along the stomach meridian and cause severe pain in this meridian, in the face, the teeth, and the eyes.

Acupuncture

The main treatment is smoothing the meridian to redistribute the wind, dissipate the heat, and improve the energy flow in the stomach meridian. The acupuncture points along the face, eyes, and teeth must be carefully selected.

The three branches of the meridian should be treated separately.

Ophthalmic nerve. This is the top branch of the trigeminal nerve. It includes Ex-HN 4 Yu Yao, GB 1 Tong Zi Liao, SJ 23 Si Zu Kong, EX-HN 5 Tai Yang, and UB 1 Jing Ming. The needles should be inserted 0.3–0.5 inches to make the patient feel a stimulation similar to an electric shock. The needles continue to be twisted three to five times and then put on the electrical stimulating machine for 30 minutes.

Maxillary nerve branch. St 2 Si Bai and St 1 Chen Qi points are used, with manipulation similar to the one used in the previous list.

Mandibular nerve branch. St 7 Xia Guan, Ren 24 Cheng Jiang, and St 4 Di Chang points are selected, with manipulation similar to one used in ophthalmic nerve. Some body points, such as GB 40 Qiu Xu, Liv 5 Li Gou, LI 4 He Gu, and Lu 7 Lie Que, are also chosen to adjust the energy of the entire body.

These acupuncture points can improve the energy flow and decrease the signal of the trigeminal nerve sent to the brain. The person must feel the sensation of the electrical shock through the practitioner's manipulation of the needles in order for the energy to flow to the trigeminal nerve to improve it and decrease the pain (see Table 13.1 and Figures 13.1 and 13.2).

Table 13.1

	Points	Meridian/ Number	Location	Conditions Helped
1	Yu Yao	EX-HN 4	At the midpoint of the eyebrow	Pain in the supraorbital region, twitching of the eyelids, drooping eyelid, cloudiness of the cornea, redness, swelling, and pain of the eye
2	Tong Zi Liao	GB 1	0.5 inches lateral to the outer canthus, in the depression on the lateral side of the orbit	Headaches, redness, and pain of the eyes, poor vision, lacrimation, deviation of the eye and mouth
3	Si Zu Kong	SJ 23	In the depression at the lateral end of the eyebrow	Headaches, redness and pain of the eye, blurring of vision, twitching of the eyelid, toothache, facial paralysis

(Continued)

Table 13.1 (*Continued*)

	Points	Meridian/ Number	Location	Conditions Helped
4	Tai Yang	EX-HN 5	In the depression about 1 inch posterior to the midpoint between the lateral end of the eyebrow and the outer canthus	Headaches, eye diseases, deviation of the eyes and mouth
5	Jing Ming	UB 1	0.1 inch superior to the inner canthus	Redness, swelling, and pain of the eye, itching of the canthus where the upper and lower eyelids meet, lacrimation, night blindness, color blindness, blurring of vision, myopia
6	Si Bai	St 2	Below St 1 in the depression at the infraorbital foramen	Redness, pain, and itching of the eye, facial paralysis, twitching of eye lids, pain in the face
7	Chen Qi	St 1	The point is directly below the pupil between the eyeball and the infraorbital ridge while the eyes are looking straight forward	Redness, swelling, and pain of the eye, lacrimation, night blindness, twitching of eyelids, facial paralysis
8	Xia Guan	St 7	At the lower border of the zygomatic arch, in the depression anterior to the condyloid process of the mandible; this point is located with the mouth closed	Deafness, tinnitus, ear discharge, toothache, facial paralysis, pain of the face, motor impairment of the jaw
9	Chen Jiang	Ren 24	In the depression of the center of the mentolabial groove	Facial puffiness, swelling of the gums, toothache, salivation, mental disorders, deviation of the eyes and mouth

(*Continued*)

Table 13.1 *(Continued)*

Points	Meridian/ Number	Location	Conditions Helped
10 Qiu Xu	GB 40	Anterior and inferior to the external malleolus, in the depression on the lateral side of the tendon of m. extensor digitorum longus	Pain in the neck, swelling in the armpit, pain in the lower abdomen, vomiting, acid regurgitation, muscular atrophy of the lower limbs, pain and swelling of the external ankle bone, malaria
11 Li Gou	Liv 5	5 inches above the tip of the medial malleolus, on the medial aspect and near the medial border of the tibia	Retention of urine, bedwetting, hernia, irregular menstruation, vaginal discharge, weakness and atrophy of the legs
12 He Gu	LI 4	On the dorsum of the hand between the 1st and 2nd metacarpal bones, approximately in the middle of the 2nd metacarpal bone on the radial side	Headaches, pain in the neck, redness, swelling, and pain of the eye, nosebleed, nasal obstruction, runny nose, toothache, deafness, swelling of the face, sore throat, salivary-gland infection, lockjaw, facial paralysis, febrile diseases with no sweating, a lot of sweating, abdominal pain, dysentery, constipation, lack of a menstrual period, delayed labor, infantile convulsions, pain, weakness, and motor impairment of the upper limbs
13 Lie Que	Lu 7	*See* Table 11.1/ Figure 12.8.	*See* Table 11.1/Figure 12.5.
14 Di Cang	St 4	Lateral to the corner of the mouth, directly below Ju Liao St 2	Deviation of the mouth, salivation, twitching of eyelids

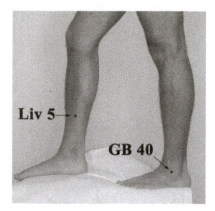

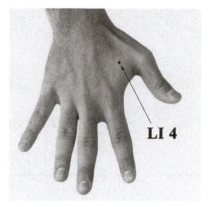

Figure 13.1   **Figure 13.2**

THOMAS'S TREATMENT

Thomas was treated with a combination of acupuncture for V2, the maxillary nerve branch, and V3, the mandibular nerve branch, plus electrical stimulation of the acupuncture needles three times a week for three weeks.

After the first visit, he felt better and reported getting a good night's sleep for the first time in six weeks. After four weeks of treatment, his pain subsided by 80 percent, so the treatments were reduced to once a month. After six months of this schedule, Thomas told me he felt no more pain.

In my experience, the treatment of this illness has two facets. First, there must be a clear diagnosis. In Thomas's case, the dentist was wrong in his evaluation of the condition and pulled two teeth unnecessarily. It is also necessary to combine Western medicine with TCM and to treat all three of the nerve branches, if necessary, though in Thomas's case two were sufficient. If this is done properly, as it was with Thomas, the person should feel much relief from the pain and be able to function normally in his or her day-to-day life.

TIPS FOR PEOPLE WITH TRIGEMINAL NEURALGIA

- Seek medical attention as early as possible.
- Using an ice-cold massage at the points mentioned in this chapter might help to decrease the pain.

TIPS FOR ACUPUNCTURE PRACTITIONERS

- In your treatment, you should combine the local points with the distal points.
- Electrical stimulation is very important.
- Do not use moxa in this case.

14

Severe Neck Pain—
Herniated Disc

Jeffrey is a 35-year-old man whose neck was affected by an automobile accident when he was rear-ended by another car as he was stopped at a red light. While he did not lose consciousness, he was aware that his neck had shifted backward, which caused only a slight pain at the time. When the police, who were called to the scene, asked him to go to the hospital for evaluation, he did not feel sufficient pain to warrant this, besides which he was due at a meeting.

About two weeks later, he noticed the neck pain was radiating down to his right shoulder, elbow, and hand, and he also felt numbness and tingling. The pain was off and on, especially during the night, and upon awakening, his neck was very stiff and painful, and he could not lift any heavy objects. At this point he visited his primary care physician, who ordered an MRI and X-ray of the neck area, and they showed a herniated disc, though no fracture, at C5 and C6. Jeffrey was referred to a neurosurgeon, who prescribed two months of physical therapy and then a follow-up visit. He began doing physical therapy three times a week, but after a few weeks the pain became worse—it was radiating not only down his right arm but also between his shoulder blades. In addition, he felt stiff and had difficulty moving his head forward and backward. The surgeon gave him a neck collar, which did not help, and suggested that, as physical therapy had not worked, he should consider surgery. Jeffrey did not want surgery. He was a self-employed car dealer and could not afford to take off the month required by surgery and recovery. He was next referred to a pain-management physician, who gave him epidural injections at C5 and C6. These made Jeffrey feel much better until a month later when the pain returned more severely than ever, and he had no idea what to do next. Fortunately, he knew someone who referred him to me for help, and after examining him, I determined that Jeffrey had cervical radiculopathy with a herniated disc.

SYMPTOMS, CAUSES, AND DIAGNOSIS

Since the cervical area, the neck, is very flexible and supports the head, it is extremely vulnerable to accidents. Car accidents, sports-related accidents, contact sports, and force can all result in different degrees of cervical injuries.

The most common neck injuries after a car accident are the following.

Soft tissue injury. This involves the muscles and ligaments. There is usually no pain radiating down to the shoulder and arm, and no numbness or tingling sensation, but the person feels neck pain on the cervical spine and posterior shoulder and experiences pain and neck weakness when he or she wakes up each morning.

Moderate to severe neck injury with a herniated disc that might impinge on the cervical nerve. The most common injury is herniated discs at C5 and C6, which impinge on the cervical nerves, causing the pain to radiate down to the shoulder, the arm, and sometimes the wrist, making the injured sides feel heavy and weak. Very often the person experiences cervical radiculopathy and feels pins and needles and a burning sensation.

Severe neck injury. This will cause a fracture or dislocation of the neck, which will, in turn, damage the spinal cord with symptoms similar to the ones mentioned earlier, but much more severe. An injury of this magnitude can very often cause paralysis.

Tests to Determine a Diagnosis

If a person feels severe neck pain after a car accident, the doctor usually orders the following tests to determine a diagnosis.

X-Rays

X-rays are the most frequently used tests, to see if there is any bone fracture. If the pain is not severe, an X-ray usually suffices.

MRI

This procedure studies the spinal cord and the nerve roots.

CT Scan

This allows a careful evaluation of the bony structure of the cervical spine.

Myelograph

This injects contrasting material into the spinal cord to evaluate both it and the nerve roots.

EMG—Electromyography

This evaluates nerve and muscle function.

TREATMENTS FOR SEVERE NECK PAIN IN WESTERN MEDICINE

Noninvasive Treatments

Depending on the test results, one or more of the following noninvasive treatments are usually given. If they are not helpful, another option is surgery.

Medications

Naproxen, Tylenol, Advil, and other anti-inflammatory drugs can be taken to decrease neck inflammation. These medications, however, just usually mask the pain, and can induce many different side effects, such as an upset stomach, a peptic ulcer, or occasionally an increased risk for a blood clot. Furthermore, they cannot be expected to specifically treat the cervical herniated disc.

Immobilization

Most people only need a soft collar, which gives psychological support to immobilize the neck and allows them to feel they can depend on it for some support. To a certain degree, this helps decrease the pain. A solid cervical orthotic might be used for an unsteady fracture of the cervical spine.

Physical Therapy

This includes heating pads, ultrasound, stretching, strengthening exercises coupled with range-of-motion exercises, and a massage. Physical therapy will help if there is soft tissue injury without a severe herniated disc. If you have a herniated disc in the neck, cervical traction

will help by slightly separating the cervical ver-
tebrae, there by allowing
the disc to gently realign
(*see* Traction).

Traction

When a person wants to
avoid surgery, the doctor
can recommend traction.
The principle of this treatment is to slightly sepa-

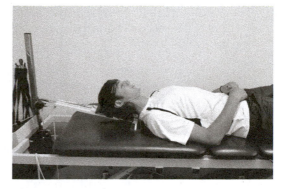

Figure 14.1

rate the vertebrae of the neck in the hope that the herniated disc might
return to its original place, thus relieving the pain. In this treatment, the
neck position is extremely important. It should not be hyperextended,
and pressure must be tested before flexing the neck, as this could cause
further damage to the cervical vertebrae (see Figure 14.1).

Invasive Treatments

Epidural Injections

With epidural injections, you are put under a specific C-arm X-ray machine, and a specially trained physician injects a steroid into the specific
herniated area and nerve root, which decreases the inflammation as well
as the pain. The treatment relies on the experience of the physician and the
severity of the herniated disc and pinched nerve. If the injury is too severe,
an epidural injection might not help, especially if the physician cannot inject the steroid into the specific point.

Surgery

If all else fails, there are two possible surgeries for this condition.

> *Discectomy.* The neurosurgeon might cut out only the herniated por-
> tion of the disc, which will relieve the pressure of the herniated disc
> on the nerve root. This may cause the symptoms to decrease or dis-
> appear.
> *Laminectomy.* Sometimes the disc degenerates or the pressure on the
> nerve root is very severe, so that removing a part of the herniated

disc is not sufficient to relieve the pain. In this case, the surgeon might cut off a piece of bone to open the nerve root outlet, which can help relieve the pain.

TREATMENTS FOR SEVERE NECK PAIN IN TRADITIONAL CHINESE MEDICINE

Jeffrey went through almost everything Western medicine could recommend, except surgery, without experiencing any significant improvement. He feared surgery and decided to consult me. After a thorough physical examination, I concluded that he had symptoms of right C5 and C6 nerve distribution, and the herniated disc was impinged at his C5 and C6 nerve roots, so I ordered an MRI of the cervical spine without contrast for Jeffrey, and it showed the following pictures (see Figure 14.2).

Acupuncture

From Figure 14.2, it is clear there was a herniated disc at C4, which impinged on the C5 nerve root and caused all the symptoms Jeffrey experienced. I employed acupuncture, following the cervical spine C5 and C6 up into the shoulder, upper arm, and forearm.

Hua Tuo Jia Ji points are sets of specially designed points used to treat disc disease. By touching the bone marker of spinal process at the worst pain points, such as C5, two needles were then inserted into 0.5 inch of the lateral sides of C5 level, one needle at the center of C5 spinal process and similarly at one level above and below at C4 and C6 level for a total of nine needles inserted about 0.5 inch deep into the herniated disc and adjacent area. (See Figure 14.3.)

I also extended the Hua Tuo Jia Ji to the C4 and C7 levels. For the other parts of body, I selected Jiang Yu, Qu Chi, Wai Guang, and He Gu. The C5 and C6 nerves go to the shoulder and upper arm, and they all follow the nerve roots. In addition, I selected the distal points, such as the bilateral Tai Chong. As I indicated in Figure 14.3, the local acupuncture points, such as Hua Tuo Jia Ji,

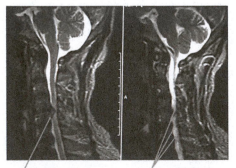

C5 Nerve Root impinged   C4, C5 and C6 Spinal
with Herniated C4 Disc   Stenosis

Figure 14.2

will increase the blood flow around that area, wash away the inflammatory factors, and decrease the muscle spasms and inflammation. The distal points, such as Tai Chong and He Gu, will greatly increase the amount of endorphins secreted into the brain, and this will decrease the pain (see Figures 14.3 to 14.5 and Table 14.1).

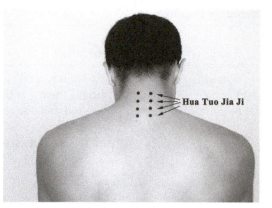

Figure 14.3

Table 14.1

	Points	Meridian/ Number	Location	Conditions Helped
1	Hua Tuo Jia Ji	Experienced Points	Along the spine, use the most painful vertebral spinal as midpoint, then locate the upper and lower spinal process, and 0.5 inches on either side, you may choose two spinal process as the starting points; *see* Figure 14.1.	Specifically treats local neck and low back pain, and pain along the spine
2	Tai Chong	Li 3	*See* Table 11.1/ Figure 11.6.	*See* Table 11.1.
3	He Gu	LI 4	*See* Table 13.1/ Figure 13.4.	*See* Table 13.1.
4	Qu Chi	LI 11	Flex the elbow, the point is in the depression of the lateral end of the transverse cubital crease	Sore throat, toothache, redness and pain of the eye, scrofula, hives, motor impairment of the upper extremities, abdominal pain, vomiting, diarrhea, febrile disease

(Continued)

Table 14.1 *(Continued)*

Points	Meridian/Number	Location	Conditions Helped
5 San Yin Jiao	Sp 6	3 inches directly above the tip of the medial malleolus, on the posterior border of the medial aspect of the tibia	Abdominal pain and distention, growling stomach, diarrhea, menstrual cramps, uterine bleeding, excessive vaginal discharge, prolapsed uterus, delayed labor, nocturnal emission, impotence, bedwetting, painful urination, swelling, hernia, pain in the external genitalia, muscular atrophy, motor impairment, paralysis and pain of the lower extremities, headaches, dizziness, vertigo, and insomnia

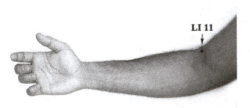

LI 11

Figure 14.4

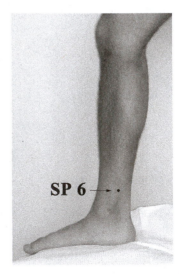

SP 6

Figure 14.5

JEFFREY'S TREATMENT

Jeffery underwent these acupuncture treatments twice a week for about 10 weeks, 20 visits in all. His pain gradually decreased, and his neck spasms and arm weakness on the right side were reduced. He now feels great improvement and is functioning normally.

TIPS FOR PEOPLE WITH SEVERE NECK PAIN

- The most effective treatment includes a combination of acupuncture, heating pads, massage, and physical therapy. Surgery is not the best option because, while there may be an improvement for about six months, the pain usually returns. After two years, many studies showed that the pain level for both surgical and nonsurgical approaches is about the same.
- It is important to seek out a clear diagnosis. For an acupuncturist to treat neck pain successfully, he or she first has to understand if the pain is moderate, requiring acupuncture treatment alone, or if it is more severe, necessitating a visit to a Western doctor. If there is a fracture, you could become paralyzed, so MRIs, X-rays, and CT scans are crucial to rule this out.

TIPS FOR ACUPUNCTURE PRACTITIONERS

- I have found that the most efficacious treatment is a combination of acupuncture, heating pads, massage, and physical therapy. I do not recommend that a patient undergo surgery immediately. Studies have shown that surgery for this condition may show a marked improvement for about six months, but after this period the pain usually returns. The pain relief period for surgery is about two years.
- A clear diagnosis is most important in these cases. For an acupuncturist to treat neck pain, he or she first has to understand the mechanism of this pain. If it is moderate, acupuncture treatment alone may help, but if it is more severe, it is important to refer the patient to a Western doctor for evaluation. If there is any fracture, the patient could become paralyzed; therefore an MRI, an X-ray, and CT scans are absolutely necessary to rule out instability.

15

Cervical Spondylosis

Andrew is a 65-year-old man who woke up one morning with neck pain, which seemingly appeared out of nowhere. He told his doctor the pain was extremely severe, shooting down from a very stiff neck to his shoulder blade. He was unable to move forward or backward and had trouble turning his neck from side to side, which made it dangerous for him to drive as he could not check to see if any cars were coming up beside him, and could not change lanes. The pain was constant, sometimes dull, sometimes sharp, but without any burning, numbness, or tingling sensation in his arms. On occasion the pain radiated up to his scalp.

Andrew's primary care physician referred him to an orthopedic doctor, who ordered an X-ray, which showed that Andrew had cervical spondylosis. He was prescribed physical therapy as his sole treatment. He went to this therapy three times a week for five weeks, which alleviated the stiffness to some degree but did nothing for the pain. He next came to me for evaluation and treatment.

SYMPTOMS, CAUSES, AND DIAGNOSIS

Cervical spondylosis is a degenerative change that affects the cervical (neck) area of the spinal cord by causing the discs and joints to compress and deteriorate between the vertebrae. It is basically arthritis of the neck and usually involves people over 40, with more men affected by it than women. The vertebrae and discs, as well as the different ligaments along the cervical spine, go through degenerative changes, with the result that you can gradually feel stiffness. When this happens, people usually try to adjust their own neck functions and flexibility, but one day when they wake up they feel very severe pain because the body can no longer adjust these positions.

The severity of symptoms depends on the location. If this compression affects the discs and ligaments, you will feel stiffness and have limitations on your range of motion; you will experience difficulty turning your head backward and forward, as well as difficulty looking over your shoulder. If the cervical nerve roots get compressed, this can cause inflammation. If you are so affected, you may feel neck pain radiating to the shoulder, and you may have urinary and bowel incontinence.

The diagnosis for this condition is based mainly on observation of the aforementioned symptoms, X-rays, and MRIs.

TREATMENTS FOR CERVICAL SPONDYLOSIS IN WESTERN MEDICINE

Noninvasive Treatments

Cervical Collars

A doctor will usually prescribe a cervical collar, normally a soft collar to start with, in order to stabilize the neck and prevent its further instability, which could lead to paralysis of the legs and or arms. If a soft collar is not sufficient, the doctor might try a more rigid neck brace. These stiff collars, however, will restrict the range of movement in the neck and may, in the long run, further exacerbate the stiffness and pain. It is not a good idea to use this method too much.

Physical Therapy

Physical therapy is another method of alleviating the condition, and it includes the use of a heating pad, electrical stimulation, ultrasound, massages, and a cervical stretch. These treatments can often be of great help (see Figures 15.1 and 15.2).

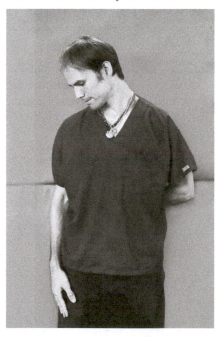

Figure 15.1

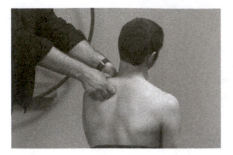

Figure 15.2

Invasive Treatments

Surgery

If the previously mentioned treatments do not work, surgery may be called for. Surgery is based on the following criteria.

- The conservative use of a cervical collar does not work.
- There is severe pain.
- There is significant neurological damage, such as difficulty raising the arm, weakness, or bladder problems.
- There is a compression of the spinal cord.

Two types of surgery are usually performed:

Laminectomy. This is a spinal operation to remove the portion of the vertebral bone called the lamina, which will release the pressure on the pinched nerves.

Discectomy. This is a surgical removal of the central portion of an intervertebral disc, the nucleus pulposus, which is causing pain by stressing the spinal cord or the radiating nerves.

Although Andrew underwent physical therapy and used a cervical collar, which provided him with some relief, he was only slightly improved, but not cured, so at this at point he consulted me for further treatment.

TREATMENTS FOR CERVICAL SPONDYLOSIS IN TRADITIONAL CHINESE MEDICINE

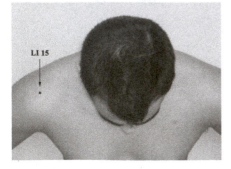

Figure 15.3

Acupuncture

The best acupuncture points for this condition are Hua Tuo Jia Ji at the C4, C5, C6, and C7, Arshi points, Du 14 Da Zhui, also LI 15 Jian Yu, LI 11 Qu Chi, SJ 5 Wai Guang, and LI 4 He Gu.

I also use small intestine meridian points, such as SI 3 Hou Xi, SI 5 Yang Gu, SI 8 Xiao Hai, SI 12 Bing Feng, and SI 11 Tian Zhong,

Table 15.1

	Points	Meridian/ Number	Location	Conditions Helped
1	Hua Tuo Jia Ji	Experience Points	Cervical, thoracic, and lumbar sacral spine; *see* Figure 14.3.	Local neck, thoracic, and low back pain
2	Arshi	Experience Points	Any tender points in the body	Decreases the pain in any tender points of the body
3	Da Zhui	Du 14	Below the spinous process of the 7th cervical vertebra, approximately at the level of the shoulders	Neck pain and rigidity, malaria, febrile diseases, epilepsy, afternoon fever, cough, asthma, common cold, back stiffness
4	Jian Yu	LI 15	Antero-inferior to the acromion, on the upper portion of m. deltoideus. When the arm is in full abduction, the point is in the depression appearing at the anterior border of the acromioclavicular joint	Pain in the shoulder and arm, motor impairment of the upper extremities, rubella, scrofula
5	Qu Chi	LI 11	*See* Table 14.1/ Figure 14.4.	*See* Table 14.1.
6	Wai Guang	SJ 5	2 inches above Yangchi between the radius and ulna	Febrile diseases, headaches, pain in the cheek, neck sprain, deafness, tinnitus, pain in the abdominal region, motor impairment of the elbow and arm, pain of the fingers, hand tremors

(Continued)

Table 15.1 *(Continued)*

	Points	Meridian/ Number	Location	Conditions Helped
7	He Gu	LI 4	*See* Table 13.1/ Figure 13.4.	*See* Table 13.1.
8	Hou Xi	SI 3	When a loose fist is made, the point is on the ulnar side, proximal to the 5th metacarpophalangeal joint, at the end of the transverse crease and the junction of the red and white skin	Pain and rigidity of the neck, tinnitus, deafness, sore throat, mania, malaria, acute lumbar sprain, night sweating, febrile diseases, contracture, and numbness of the fingers, pain in the shoulder and elbow
9	Yang Gu	SI 5	At the ulnar end of the transverse crease on the dorsal aspect of the wrist, in the depression between the styloid process of the ulna and triquetral bone	Swelling of the neck and jaw region, pain of the hand and wrist, febrile diseases
10	Xiao Hai	SI 8	When the elbow is flexed, the point is located in the depression between the olecranon of the ulna and the medial epicondyle of the humerus	Headaches, swelling of the cheek, pain in the neck, shoulder, arm, and elbow, epilepsy
11	Bing Feng	SI 12	In the center of the suprascapular fossa, directly above Tian Zhong; when the arm is lifted, the point is at the site of the depression	Pain in the scapular region, numbness, and aching of the upper extremities, motor impairment of the shoulder and arm

(Continued)

Table 15.1 (*Continued*)

	Points	Meridian/ Number	Location	Conditions Helped
12	Tian Zhong	SI 11	In the infrascapular fossa, at the junction of the upper and middle third of the distance between the lower border of the scapular spine and the inferior angle of the scapula	Pain in the scapular region of the back, and in the elbow and arm, asthma

to balance the energy of the entire upper extremity (see Table 15.1 and Figures 15.3 to 15.6).

It is important to bear in mind that acupuncture alone cannot cure spondylosis because degenerative changes of the cervical spine severely affect both the ligaments and the joints. In people older than 40, calcium often starts to break loose from the bones and circulate in the blood flow. This circulated calcium begins to affect the different joints, and if it does so on the cervical spine, it will cause the deterioration in the ligaments, discs, and joints known as cervical spondylosis and will restrict range of

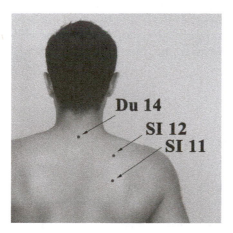

Figure 15.4

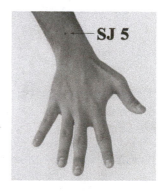

Figure 15.5

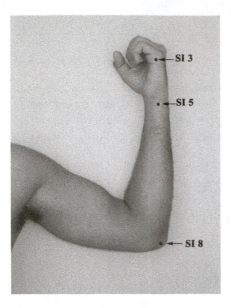

motion in the neck. Acupuncture may help relieve some of the symptoms, mainly pain, but the physical degeneration is unlikely to be helped by this method.

Since this condition is ongoing, and can cause difficulty walking, numbness, a tingling sensation in the arms and hands, weakness of the arms, and urinary tract incontinence, the earlier it is treated, the better. These symptoms can become dangerous, causing permanent loss of nerve function, and in this case, surgery will be absolutely necessary; the sooner, the better.

Figure 15.6

ANDREW'S TREATMENT

I first treated Andrew for his cervical spondylosis by placing a heating pad on his neck for 15 minutes and then inserting the acupuncture needles at the points listed earlier. The acupuncture was coupled with strong electrical stimulation, after which Andrew was treated with ultrasound and a massage. After six weeks of treatment, his neck function was much improved, and he was again able to turn his head without difficulty when he was driving. He was therefore able to avoid surgery, and while he still experienced minimal pain, the acupuncture was able to help his condition and strengthen the main function of his cervical spine.

TIPS FOR PEOPLE WITH CERVICAL SPONDYLOSIS

- Using a heating pad will help healing.
- You may accompany the acupuncture treatment with a massage and range-of-motion exercises for your neck.

TIPS FOR ACUPUNCTURE PRACTITIONERS

- Before inserting the needles, always put a heating pad on the patient's neck for about 15 minutes. The heating pad will improve circulation.
- Hua Tuo Jia Ji is an excellent group of acupuncture points you should always use for your patient's neck pain.

16

Acute Neck Spasms

Harry, a 26-year-old man, came to me complaining of neck pain and stiffness. Five days before the visit, he had ordered a new mattress, which he tried to move into his apartment, carrying it on his shoulder and neck. When he got it into the apartment, his neck went into spasm and he was not able to move it at all. He subsequently experienced difficulty sleeping and could not bend forward or backward, or turn his neck, even to a 10-degree angle. He could barely move and felt very frustrated, especially as he was to get married one day after first consulting me.

After examining Harry, I concluded he had no neurological injury. Though the pain had radiated down his arm, he had no weakness. His only symptom was the tightness in his neck and his inability to bend forward or backward, or turn his head. I determined that Harry was experiencing an acute muscle spasm—he had carried the mattress for his new, post-wedding home on his back and neck, and this pushed his neck forward suddenly, causing the muscle spasm.

SYMPTOMS, CAUSES, AND DIAGNOSIS

An acute muscle spasm can be caused by different movements, such as cradling the phone against the neck when making a call, hoisting groceries out of the car, or waking up with neck pain after sleeping in an awkward position. When a muscle spasms, all the fibrous material within the core of the muscle contracts simultaneously. Quickly bending over after sitting can overstretch the neck and back muscles and injure that area. In response to this spasm, the surrounding muscle fibers tighten, forming a protective splint to guard against further irritation, which triggers a painful backstabbing cycle. A contracted squeeze of blood flow to the muscles causes irritation and more pain, and this additional pain triggers an even tighter contraction.

The diagnosis for this condition is based on clinical findings, such as neck pain, difficulty bending or turning around, a fall, or an accident. X-rays are not needed to make the diagnosis.

TREATMENTS FOR ACUTE NECK SPASMS IN WESTERN MEDICINE

Noninvasive Treatments

For treatments in Western medicine, the following methods are usually employed.

- Lying on a bed and bringing your knees up to your chin. This often relieves the muscle spasm.
- A gentle ice massage decreases the blood flow to the spasm, which forces the muscle fibers to relax.
- Anti-inflammatory medication, such as ibuprofen, is used, which may or may not help.

TREATMENTS FOR ACUTE NECK SPASMS IN TRADITIONAL CHINESE MEDICINE

Acupuncture

For this acute problem, I use SI 3 Hou Xi, GB 39 Jue Gu, Arshi, and Luo Zhen, which is an experienced point specifically for acute neck sprain, and ancillary points, such as Du 14 Da Zhui, GB 20 Feng Chi, UB 10 Tian Zhu, UB 60 Kun Lun, and UB 11 Da Zhu.

Other beneficial treatment options include a massage, a heating pad, and a foam roller. Using the foam roller from the bottom to the top of the shoulder blades for two minutes, as shown in Table 16.1 and Figures 16.1 to 16.6 can assist in relaxing the muscle spasm.

HARRY'S TREATMENT

Before consulting me, Harry had tried all the Western treatments, and at this point I decided to use acupuncture. I treated him with the previously mentioned points for 20 minutes and then gave him a treatment with a heating pad and a massage, after which I stretched his neck and back muscles.

Table 16.1

	Points	Meridian/Number	Location	Conditions Helped
1	Hou Xi	SI 3	*See* Table 15.1/Figure 15.6	*See* Table 15.1
2	Jue Gu (Xuan Zhong)	GB 39	3 inches above the tip of the external malleolus, in the depression between the posterior border of the fibula and tendons of m. peroneal longus and brevis	Apoplexy, paralysis on one side, neck pain, abdominal distension, pain in the abdomen, muscular atrophy of the lower limbs, spastic pain of the leg, beriberi
3	Arshi	Experience Points	Any tender points in the body	Decreased pain in the body
4	Lao Zhen	Experience Point	Back of the palm between the 2nd and 3rd MCP joints, 1 inch proximal to the MCP joints	Decreased spasm of the neck muscles
5	Da Zhui	Du 14	*See* Table 5.1/Figure 5.4.	*See* Table 5.1.
6	Feng Chi	GB 20	*See* Table 11.1/Figure 11.5.	*See* Table 11.1.
7	Tian Zhu	UB 10	1.3 inches lateral to Ya Men (Du 15), in the depression on the lateral aspect of m. trapezius	Headaches, nasal obstruction, sore throat, neck rigidity, pain in the shoulder and back
8	Kun Lun	UB 60	In the depression between the external malleolus and tendon calcaneus	Headaches, blurring of vision, neck rigidity, nosebleed, pain in the shoulder, back, and arm, swelling and pain in the heel, difficult labor, epilepsy
9	Da Zhu	UB 11	1.5 inches lateral to Tao Dao (Du 13), at the level of the lower border of the spinous process of the 1st thoracic vertebra	Headaches, pain in the neck, back, and scapular region, cough, fever, neck rigidity

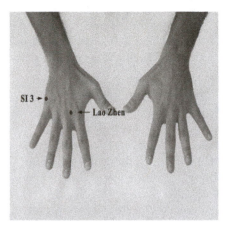

Figure 16.1

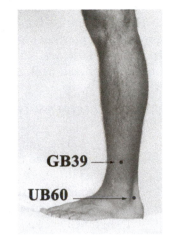

Figure 16.2

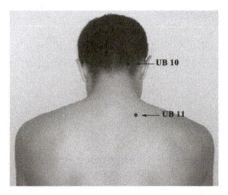

Figure 16.3

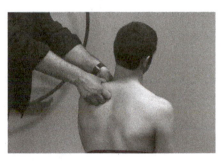

Figure 16.4

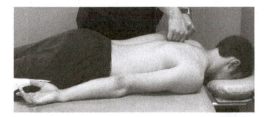

Figure 16.5

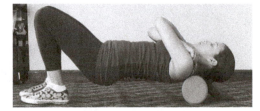

Figure 16.6

Harry felt immediate relief on this crucial first visit and came in for another treatment before his wedding the next day. After the additional treatment, Harry was able to go through the wedding and reception without any restricted neck movement.

TIPS FOR PEOPLE WITH ACUTE NECK SPASMS

- If you cannot find an acupuncturist immediately, do not panic. Put a heating pad on your neck for 20 minutes, then press the Lao Zhen point (see Figure 16.1) for about 20 minutes, and then try to move your neck around. This will usually work.
- If it does not work, try alternating a cold pad with a heating pad, 15 minutes for each, and then repeat the above acupressure.

TIPS FOR ACUPUNCTURE PRACTITIONERS

- Insert one needle about 0.5 inches into the Lao Zhen point slightly upward to the wrist and elbow, twist the needle strongly, and make the patient feel the electrical sensation radiating to the arm and shoulder. Next, insert one needle to SI 3, twist it, and make the electrical sensation radiate to the little fingertip. In the meantime, ask the patient to turn his or her neck around. The patient will usually feel an immediate relief of the neck spasm.
- If the previously mentioned methods do not induce a good response and do not release the pain, you may insert one needle about one inch to GB 39 toward the knee, then strongly twist it, and ask the patient turn his or her neck.
- You may add moxa, a type of burning herbs wrapped around a needle, to accelerate the recovery.

17

Frozen Shoulder

Martha is a 50-year-old woman with a long history of diabetes. Several months back, she felt a slight pain in her right shoulder upon lifting a heavy object that caused her to drop it. Though the pain was not too bad for a few weeks, she gradually noticed that the shoulder was working less and less and was becoming extremely painful. She had trouble lifting her arms to do such simple tasks as combing her hair or dressing with ease, and putting clothes on her right arm or fastening her brassiere became increasingly difficult. Hoping the pain would go away on its own, she did not consult a doctor until the pain became so severe that she came to me.

In examining Martha, I found there was moderate tenderness at the front and back of her right shoulder, upper arm, and elbow. She had difficulty raising her right shoulder up to her head or across the middle of her body and said that she was unable to sleep on her right side. The pain was constant and caused weakness in her right arm. There was no numbness or tingling sensation. I determined that Martha probably had a frozen shoulder, the medical term for which is *adhesive capsulitis*.

SYMPTOMS, CAUSES, AND DIAGNOSIS

This condition usually occurs after age 40, and about 20 percent of those who experience the disorder have a history of diabetes with, for most, a history of accidents as well. When these people start to feel shoulder pain, they try to compensate by lessening the movements of the injured shoulder, but this leads to limiting the range of motion for the shoulder, which makes some normal tasks, such as brushing hair, dressing, and reaching up high, more difficult. By the time it reaches this stage, the person realizes it is necessary to seek medical treatment for this condition.

Frozen shoulder usually has three stages.

Painful stage. This comes on gradually, and there is vague pain that lasts about eight months (without knowing any specific date of onset.)

Frozen stage. The pain may begin to diminish during this stage, but the shoulder becomes stiffer and the range of motion decreases noticeably, which causes the person to avoid extreme movements that exacerbate the pain. This phase usually lasts from six weeks to nine months.

Thawing stage. During this stage that can last from five months to two years, the shoulder movement gradually returns to normal, and the pain lessens.

The causes of frozen shoulder are still unclear, though the following possibilities are noted.

- Frozen shoulder can be caused by an injury resulting from surgery or by any trauma accident. Most people who develop this condition have a history of injury, which causes pain and a decrease in the range of movements.
- People with diabetes tend to develop frozen shoulder (about 20% of those affected). For them, diabetes worsens their symptoms.
- Autoimmune or inflammatory conditions and any procedures that immobilize the shoulder will increase the chances of developing a frozen shoulder.

This condition is diagnosed by an examination of the shoulder to determine if there has been a significant reduction (at least 50%) in both active and passive range of motion. X-rays can also be done to rule out a fracture, an underlying tumor, or calcium deposits. MRIs are necessary if the person's pain and range of motion has not improved after three months of treatment.

TREATMENTS FOR FROZEN SHOULDER IN WESTERN MEDICINE

Noninvasive Treatments

Medications

The use of anti-inflammatory medications, such as ibuprofen or naproxen, is widespread, but taking these medications by mouth is not considered very effective.

Physical Therapy

This treatment involves a heating pad, stretching, wheel range of motion (see Figures 17.1, to 17.3), muscle strengthening, electrical stimulation, ultrasound, electrophoresis (electrical current used to deliver topical corticosteroid medications through your skin), or dual treatments—injections plus physical therapy, which can be very effective.

Invasive Treatments

Injections

Using corticosteroids, such as 40 mg of Kenalog and 5 cc of lidocaine injected directly into the shoulder bursa, will greatly decrease the intensity

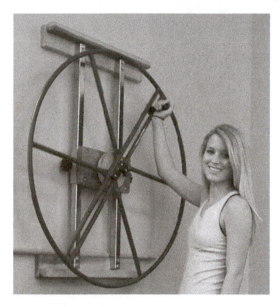

Figure 17.1

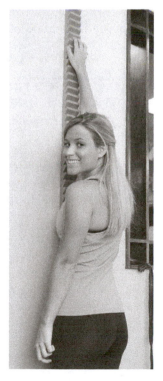

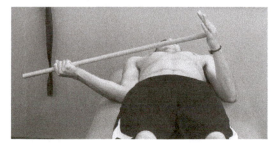

Figure 17.2

Figure 17.3

of pain. However, there are some negative side effects of corticosteroid injections, such as elevated blood sugar, a fragile shoulder tendon, or osteoporosis. Unless absolutely necessary, I do not usually recommend using corticosteroid injections in such cases as severe pain, a largely decreased range of motion, or a marked containment of normal daily activities.

Surgery

In some cases surgical treatment may be necessary.

> *Manipulation under general anesthesia* is one procedure. This forces the shoulder to move, but the downside is that the process can cause the capsule in the shoulder to stretch or tear.
>
> *Shoulder arthroscopy.* In this type of surgery, the doctor makes several small incisions around the shoulder capsule. A minute camera and instrument are inserted through the incision, and the instrument is used to cut through the tight portion of the joint capsule.

Manipulation and arthroscopic surgeries are often used together, and many have good results with this type of surgery (see Figures 17.1 to 17.3).

TREATMENTS FOR FROZEN SHOULDER IN TRADITIONAL CHINESE MEDICINE

Acupuncture

The following points are selected for frozen shoulder: LI 15 Jian Yu, SI 9 Jian Zhen, SJ 14 Jian Liao, SI 10 Nao Shu, SI 11 Tian Zhong, LI 16 Ju Gu, St 38 Tiao Kou penetrating to UB 57 Cheng Shan, SJ 5 Wai Guan, LI 4 He Gu, and LI 11 Qu Chi (see Table 17.1 and Figures 17.4 to 17.7).

MARTHA'S TREATMENT

I put a heating pad on Martha's right shoulder for about 20 minutes so the tendon underneath the heating pad would start to be more flexible; then I inserted the needles into the acupuncture points mentioned earlier. After 30 minutes of acupuncture treatment, deep massage was given, along with range-of-motion exercises, after which Martha was able to

Table 17.1

	Points	Meridian/ Number	Location	Conditions Helped
1	Jian Qian	Experienced Points	Anterior to the shoulder joint, at the origin of bicipital tendon	Biceps tendonitis, frozen shoulder
2	Jian Yu	LI 15	*See* Table 15.1/ Figure 15.3.	*See* Table 15.1.
3	Jian Zhen	SI 9	Posterior and inferior to the shoulder joint. When the arm is adducted, the point is 1 inch above the posterior end of the axillary fold	Pain in the scapular region, motor impairment of the head and arm
4	Jian Liao	SJ 14	Posterior and inferior to the acromion, in the depression about 1 inch posterior to LI 15, Jian Yu, when the arm is abducted	Pain and motor impairment of the shoulder and upper arm
5	Nao Shu	SI 10	When the arm is adducted, the point is directly above SI 9, Jian Zhen, in the depression inferior to the scapular spine	Swelling of the shoulder, aching and weakness of the shoulder and arm
6	Tian Zhong	SI 11	*See* Table 15.1 / Figure 15.4.	*See* Table 15.1.
7	Ju Gu	LI 16	In the upper aspect of the shoulder, in the depression between the acromial extremity of the clavicle and the scapular spine	Pain and motor impairment of the upper extremities, pain in the shoulder and back

(Continued)

Table 17.1   (*Continued*)

	Points	Meridian/ Number	Location	Conditions Helped
8	Tian Kou	St 38	2 inches below St 37, Shang Ju Xu, midway between St 35 Du Bi and St 41 Jie Xi.	Numbness, soreness, and pain in the knee and leg, weakness and motor impairment of the foot, pain and motor impairment of the shoulder, abdominal pain
9	Cheng Shan	UB 57	Directly below the belly of m. gastrocnemius, on the line joining UB 40 Wei Zhong and tendo calcaneus, about 8 inches below UB 40	Low back pain, spasm of the big calf muscle at the back of the lower leg, hemorrhoids, constipation, beriberi
10	Wai Guan	SJ 5	*See* Table 15.1/Figure 15.5.	*See* Table 15.1.
11	He Gu	LI 4	*See* Table 13.1/Figure 13.4.	*See* Table 13.1.
12	Qu Chi	LI 11	*See* Table 14.1/Figure 14.4.	*See* Table 14.1.

successfully raise her shoulder. She underwent my treatment for a total of 10 visits and reported that her right shoulder pain and her range of motion were much improved.

TIPS FOR PEOPLE WITH FROZEN SHOULDER

- Do range-of-motion exercises for 20 minutes every morning after a hot bath or shower. This is to increase your blood circulation and

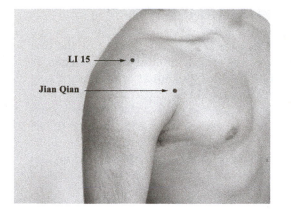

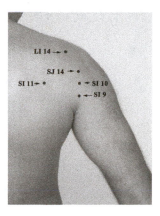

Figure 17.4

Figure 17.5

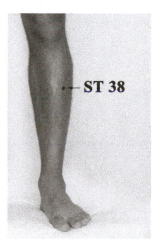

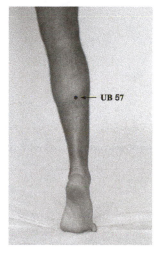

Figure 17.6

Figure 17.7

energy flow after the hot water on the shoulder, and it will lead to the least pain and best range of motion.

- Purchase a heating pad, apply heat on the shoulder for 20 minutes, and then do range-of-motion exercises, which will improve your shoulder mobility.
- The main goal is to increase the range of motion of the shoulder, and the second goal is to decrease the pain on the shoulder.
- Try to get treatment ASAP. Do not wait. If you wait, it may take a few years for natural recovery or you may not recover any range of motion at all.

TIPS FOR ACUPUNCTURE PRACTITIONERS

- Have the patients seated in a relaxed position and put the first needle in Qu Chi tips toward the shoulder, about 1.5 inches, to make the energy transmit to the shoulder, and then insert the needles into the Jian Yu, Jian Zhen, Jian Liao, and Tian Zhong points, also the Tiao Kou point penetrating to Cheng Shan. In the meantime, scratch the handles of the needles and ask the patient to feel the energy from the needle tips spreading to the shoulder.
- Tell your patient to slowly raise his or her arm up to the head, and move the arm around. The patient will usually feel a degree of instant relief from the pain.

18

Rotator Cuff Tendonitis

Arnold, a 45-year-old man, was playing with his young son and pitched him a few baseballs, after which he felt a sudden onset of right shoulder pain that was so severe he could not raise his arm or reach up. Needless to say, this interfered considerably with his daily activities.

When I questioned Arnold, he told me he had had this pain off and on for more than six months, but it was mild enough that he did not feel it was necessary to see a doctor. His pain radiated from the front of the shoulder to the side of the arm and was present during both day and night activities. Lately, he told me, the pain had been getting steadily worse, but because his son had recently returned from boarding school, he was anxious to play baseball with him, which no doubt worsened his condition as he was no longer able to raise his arm to 90 degrees. When I performed the physical examination, I realized Arnold's right shoulder was moderately swollen and very tender to the touch at the front and back of the deltoid area, and the arch between 60 and 120 degrees was painful. I had to help him raise his arm from 60 to 90 degrees, which caused him pain, but once he got it past the 120-degree mark, he could do it himself and the pain subsided. I also tried a drop-arm test in which I lifted his right arm up passively to 90 degrees, then let it go, and he had difficulty maintaining the arm at this position on his own. Based on the these observations, I determined that Arnold had most likely torn his rotator cuff.

SYMPTOMS, CAUSES, AND DIAGNOSIS

Rotator cuff tendonitis has different names, including rotator cuff inflammation, shoulder impingement syndrome, and rotator cuff bursitis. The common symptom is that people experience a gradual onset of shoulder pain and have difficulty raising their arms up to 120 degrees. Impingement of the rotator cuff tendons is the most common cause of shoulder pain.

The rotator cuff is a group of tendons composed of four muscles: the supraspinatus, infraspinatus, teres minor, and subscapularis. These muscles cover the head of the humerus, and along with the deltoid muscle, they form the bow of the shoulder. The function of these muscles is to rotate and lift the shoulder.

The front edge of the shoulder is called the acromion. It sits over and in front of the humeral head when the arm is lifted and, in most cases, will not rub the tendons of the rotator cuff. However, in some cases the acromion might wrap, or impinge on, the surface of the rotator cuff, which causes pain and limits the shoulder movement. This is called impingement syndrome, and there are three stages to it:

> *Stage One—Edema or hemorrhage stage.* This usually occurs in people under age 25. The shoulder shows acute pain, edema, or hemorrhage, with signs of inflammation. This stage is reversible and surgery usually is not the option.
>
> *Stage Two—Fibrosis and tendonitis stage.* The inflamed rotator cuff tendons continue to get worse and develop into fibrosis and tendonitis. This most often occurs between age 25 and 40. Depending on the person's condition, both conservative treatment and surgery should be considered.
>
> *Stage Three.* Acromioclavicular spur and rotator cuff tear will progress from stage two, and surgical repair is commonly required.

Arnold appeared to have stage three, a rotator cuff tear, but in order to make a clear diagnosis, I ordered X-rays. They showed a large anterior spur, which caused the impingement of the rotator cuff and the pain. When Arnold played ball with his son, he traumatized his shoulder and caused the rotator cuff to tear.

TREATMENTS FOR ROTATOR CUFF SYNDROME IN WESTERN MEDICINE

Noninvasive Treatments

Western medicine divides noninvasive treatment three ways. Many people experience gradual improvement and return to normal function with these methods.

Medications

A course of oral prednisone or some nonsteroidal anti-inflammatory drugs is given.

Ice Packs

Strenuous activity is to be avoided, and an ice pack is put on the injured shoulder.

Physical Therapy

This can take from several weeks to a number of months.

Stretching tight structures of the shoulder, such as the sleeper stretch, can be performed a few times daily. In this stretch, you bring the bottom arm down to the table with the assistance of the top arm, hold that pose for 10 seconds, and repeat it five times.

External rotation of the shoulder is a great strengthening exercise for the rotator cuff and should be done in up to three sets of 10 reps (see Figures 18.1 to 18.4).

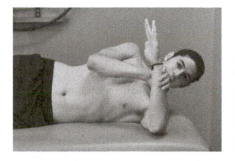

Figure 18.1   Start

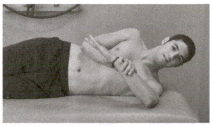

Figure 18.2   Finish

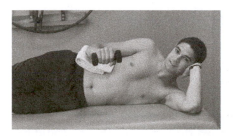

Figure 18.3   Start

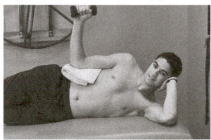

Figure 18.4   Finish

Invasive Treatments

Injections

A steroid is injected into the affected area.

Surgery

Surgical treatment is usually indicated for full thickness, an entire layer, or partial rotator cuff tendon tears that failed conservative treatment.

There are two kinds of surgical techniques:

Arthroscopic technique. Two or three small puncture wounds are made in the shoulder, and a small instrument is inserted to reshape the surface of the acromion and clean out the injured tissue of the rotator cuff.

Open technique. Open surgery is performed to cut open the shoulder and then directly visualize the acromion and rotator cuff to determine the next step of treatment. If it is necessary, the surgeon may reshape the acromion or sew the torn rotator cuff tendons.

TREATMENTS FOR ROTATOR CUFF SYNDROME IN TRADITIONAL CHINESE MEDICINE

Acupuncture

In my acupuncture treatment, I use *"the three famous shoulder needles,"* Jian Qian, Jian Yu, and Jian Zhen. All these must be inserted 2–3 inches into specific anatomical points in the rotator cuff—the bicipital, the supraspinatus tendons, and the acromial bursa—and be followed by strong electrical stimulation. This brings a large amount of blood flow to the shoulder and washes away the inflammation, which gradually diminishes the sensation of pain and improves the range of shoulder motion.

The ancillary points include LI 14 Bi Nao, SJ 5 Wai Guan, LI 4 He Gu, and LI 11 Qu Chi (see Table 18.1).

ARNOLD'S TREATMENT

Arnold was offered all the Western options, including surgery, but because he was a busy businessman who supplied flowers globally and could not afford to lose any time from work, he opted for conservative treatment. In

Table 18.1

	Points	Meridian/ Number	Location	Conditions Helped
1	Jian Qian	Extra 23	Anterior to the shoulder joint, at the origin of bicipital tendon	Biceps tendonitis, frozen shoulder
2	Jian Yu	LI 15	Antero-inferior to the acromion, on the upper portion of m. deltoideus; when the arm is in full abduction, the point is in the depression appearing at the anterior border of the acromioclavicular joint	Pain in the shoulder and arm, motor impairment of the upper extremities, German measles, scrofula
3	Jian Zhen	SI 9	Posterior and inferior to the shoulder joint; when the arm is adducted, the point is 1 inch above the posterior end of the axillary fold	Pain in the region of the scapula, motor impairment of the hand and arm
4	Bi Nao	LI 14	On the line joining Qu Chi (LI 11) and Jian Yu (LI 15), 7 inches above Qu Chi (LI 11), on the radial side of the humerus, superior to the lower end of the m. deltoideus	Pain in the shoulder and arm, rigidity of the neck, scrofula
5	Wai Guan	SJ 5	*See* Table 15.1/ Figure 15.5.	*See* Table 15.1.
6	He Gu	LI 4	*See* Table 13.1/ Figure 13.4.	*See* Table 13.1.
7	Qu Chi	LI11	*See* Table 14.1/ Figure 14.4.	*See* Table 14.1.

his case, I combined physical therapy with acupuncture. I advised him to put an ice pack on his shoulder immediately and to rest his arm as much as possible, strictly avoiding any activities that might aggravate the symptoms. I then introduced acupuncture to decrease the pain. I treated Arnold for about three months, and after he passed through the acute stage, I was able to gradually strengthen his rotator cuff muscle. After six months, his shoulder and his range of motion returned to normal, so there was no need for surgery. With his tendonitis much improved, he was happy to again be able to throw a ball with his son without experiencing pain.

TIPS FOR PEOPLE WITH ROTATOR CUFF TENDONITIS

- If you have rotator cuff tendonitis that is in the acute stage and you are less than age 25, putting an ice pack on the shoulder helps decrease the swelling and inflammation.
- For stage two fibrosis and tendonitis, if you are between 25 and 40 years old, acupuncture, as described earlier, should be started as soon as possible. At this stage, this is usually sufficient treatment.
- The stage three condition, the acromioclavicular spur and rotator cuff tear, usually occurs if you are 40 or older. X-rays and an MRI are advised, as is a visit to an orthopedic surgeon to see if surgery is indicated. If you are young and the injury is sports-related, suturing the torn rotator cuff as soon as possible can help speed up a complete recovery.

TIPS FOR ACUPUNCTURE PRACTITIONERS

- If your patient has rotator cuff tendonitis or impingement, and is less than 25 years old and in the acute stage, an ice pack on the shoulder to decrease both the edema and inflammation, followed by acupuncture, is usually a sufficient cure.
- For stage two fibrosis and tendonitis that usually occurs between ages 25 and 40, acupuncture should start as soon as possible. This is usually sufficient treatment at this stage.
- Stage three, the acromioclavicular spur and rotator cuff tear condition, usually occurs in patients over 40. In this case, treatment should be extremely cautious and the patient should have an X-ray and MRI without contrast, to discover if there is a partial or complete tear, and should consult an orthopedic surgeon as well, to see if surgery is indicated. If the patient is young and the injury is related to sports, the torn rotator cuff should be sutured as soon as possible in order to accelerate a complete recovery.

19

Shoulder Arthritis

Brittany, a 65-year-old woman, experienced on-and-off pain in her shoulder for two or three years, especially upon awakening. The pain was located on the front, sometimes the top, of her shoulder, which made everyday tasks, such as reaching for a high shelf or combing her hair, difficult for her. It also caused swelling of her right shoulder, which became worse when the weather changed, so much so that she told her friends she was a human weathervane. Recently, she began to feel a clicking or grinding sound in the shoulder, and it became increasingly difficult for her to fall or stay asleep due to the pain, which had been increasing for several years.

Brittany was a basketball player in college, and sometimes when she shot the ball, she felt some pain, but it went away after a day or two. She began taking Tylenol and Advil, which gave some relief, but because she was so occupied with her own business, and because she always assumed the pain would eventually go away, she never made the time to go to a doctor before she came to me.

In my physical exam, I found the deltoid muscle of her right shoulder was atrophied. The right shoulder front, top, and back of the shoulder blade were all tender. When I performed a range-of-motion test, the flexing in the right shoulder was about 0–120 degrees and her extension was about 0–115 degrees, with pain in the 0- to 70-degree extension. The grinding, cracking noise that accompanied this extension made the pain in this shoulder feel worse, but I found no signs of arthritis in other joints, including the left shoulder, which was perfectly normal.

SYMPTOMS, CAUSES, AND DIAGNOSIS

There are two main shoulder joints that can develop one of the three main types of arthritis.

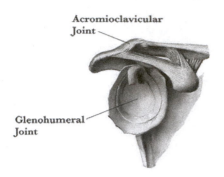

Figure 19.1

The glenohumeral joint (also called the bone-circuit joint). Here, the typical pain is on the top and back of the shoulder, and it sometimes involves pain in the shoulder blade, the scapula, and restricted range of motion.

The acromioclavicular joint. Arthritis can develop where the collarbone meets the shoulder blade (scapula), at the bony prominence on the top of the shoulder blade known as the acromion. The pain is at the top of the shoulder and increases when, for example, the arm is crossed in front of the body to touch the other shoulder, or the arm is raised to comb the hair or take something from a high shelf (see Figure 19.1).

There are three principal types of arthritis that can affect the shoulder:

Osteoarthritis, inflammation of the joints, is caused by wear and tear, and the diagnosis is made by X-rays and observing the symptoms.

Rheumatoid arthritis, an autoimmune disease that is usually a symmetrical inflammation of the joints, especially the shoulder, knee, and other small joints. The diagnosis is based on blood work, such as positive rheumatoid factors, observing symptoms, and X-rays.

Posttraumatic arthritis, which results from injury. The diagnosis is determined by a history of the trauma and X-ray changes.

TREATMENTS FOR SHOULDER ARTHRITIS IN WESTERN MEDICINE

Noninvasive Treatments

The first methods to try are the nonsurgical treatments.

Rest

Rest and changing physical activities. The patient should avoid any activity that provokes pain.

Compresses

Using hot and cold compresses can be very helpful.

Physical Therapy

Physical therapy and massages. The following are a few exercises that will help strengthen the rotator cuff to allow more fluid motion. Three sets of 10 each should be performed three times a week (see Figures 19.2 and 19.3).

Invasive Treatment

Surgery

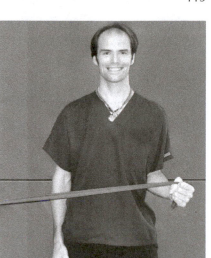

Figure 19.2

If nonsurgical treatments do not work, then surgery would be necessary.

Resection arthroplasty is the most common surgical procedure for arthritis of the acromioclavicular joint. Its purpose is to restore the flexible connection between the acromion and the collarbone. A small piece of bone from the end of the collarbone is removed, leaving a space that later fills in with scar tissue.

Total shoulder arthroplasty for glenohumeral joint arthritis. In this procedure, a surgeon replaces the entire shoulder joint with a prosthesis.

Hemiarthroplasty, also for glenohumeral joint arthritis. In this procedure, the surgeon replaces the head of the upper arm bone. One joint surface is replaced with an artificial material, usually metal.

I suggest to most of my patients that they try nonsurgical treatments first. However, if the pain is intolerable and severely restricts sleep, a surgical treatment might be the better of the two options.

Figure 19.3

TREATMENTS FOR SHOULDER ARTHRITIS IN TRADITIONAL CHINESE MEDICINE

Acupuncture

When performed appropriately, acupuncture can help with two types of osteoarthritis.

For glenohumeral osteoarthritis, I use LI 15 Jian Yu, SJ 14 Jian Liao, SI 9 Jian Zhen, LI11 Qu chi, LI4 He Gu, and also SI 11 Tian Zhong and Extra Points 23 Jian Qian. All needles need to be inserted to about 1.5 inches with electrical stimulation for about 30 minutes. The patient must be in a seated position and the electrical stimulation should be as high as can be tolerated.

For acromioclavicular osteoarthritis, it is essential to locate the exact point of tenderness in the front of the shoulder and the AC joint and insert the needle into that AC joint and then the remaining points as in the preceding paragraph. This principle of treatment is called *acupuncture points selection based on the pain location,* aka the specific anatomical location following the pain points (see Table 19.1).

Table 19.1

	Points	Meridian/ Number	Location	Conditions Helped
1	Jian Qian	Extra Points 23	*See* Table 18.1/Figure 18.5.	*See* Table 18.1.
2	Jian Yu	LI 15	*See* Table 18.1/Figure 18.5.	*See* Table 18.1.
3	Jian Zhen	SI 9	*See* Table 18.1/Figure 18.5.	*See* Table 18.1.
4	Jian Liao	SJ 14	*See* Table 17.1/Figure 17.5.	*See* Table 17.1.
5	Qu Chi	LI 11	*See* Table 14.1/Figure 14.4.	*See* Table 14.1.
6	Tian Zhong	SI 11	*See* Table 15.1/Figure 15.4.	*See* Table 15.1.
7	Wai Guan	SJ 5	*See* Table 15.1/Figure 15.5.	*See* Table 15.1.
8	He Gu	LI 4	*See* Table 13.1/Figure 13.4.	*See* Table 13.1.

BRITTANY'S TREATMENT

Brittany had an X-ray that showed the cartilage of her right shoulder was wearing out. On the glenohumeral joint, there was a loss of joint space and bone spurs were present. She was also given a blood test to rule out rheumatoid arthritis, and it came back negative.

Brittany was advised to avoid lifting anything heavy, stop using weights, or doing any other upper-extremity exercises, including basketball, if she still played that sport.

If her shoulder was swollen, Brittany was advised to use a cold pad for 15–20 minutes three times a day; conversely, if there was no swelling; then she was advised to use a heating pad in the same manner. Acupuncture, physical therapy, and massage were to be tried before any surgery was performed.

Brittany received treatment three times a week for six to eight weeks, and her shoulder pain was much relieved. However, I had to advise her that acupuncture cannot change the lost cartilage or remove the clicking, snapping sound. It could decrease the pain, making it improved enough that she would be able to get a good night's sleep and could prolong the need for surgery. Brittany reported that this was indeed the case after the treatments. Her pain diminished enough to allow her to go on living her life without having to resort to surgery. She survived for three years without surgery, which gave her a comfortable level of living.

TIPS FOR PEOPLE WITH SHOULDER OSTEOARTHRITIS

- If your shoulder is a normal temperature, always put a heating pad on it twice a day for 30 minutes each time. If it is hot, place a cold pad there for the same amount of time.
- After the hot or cold pad, spend 30 minutes a day doing range-of-motion exercises for the shoulder. These will greatly improve your shoulder mobility and decrease the pain.

TIPS FOR ACUPUNCTURE PRACTITIONERS

- Before an acupuncture treatment, you should always check the temperature of the shoulder. If it is hot, place a cold pad on the shoulder for at least 15 minutes; if it is normal body temperature, place a heating pad there for 15 minutes or more.

- For glenohumeral osteoarthritis, the needles should be inserted at least about 1.5 inches deep; for acromioclavicular osteoarthritis, insert the needles about 1 inch deep.
- Treat with electrical stimulation for 20–30 minutes. You might want to tell your patients that the pain could increase a bit but will subside after a few treatments.

20

Bilateral Elbow Pain

Christina, 25 years old, is a recent graduate of music school where her instrument was the violin. With a large tuition loan to repay, Christina teaches 30–40 students a day in group lessons, but not long ago she started feeling pain in the left lateral and medial elbow. The pain, which radiated from the inside of the elbow into the forearm and wrist, was constant, and she experienced it whenever she played her violin. When she flexed her wrist, the pain worsened and she experienced weakness in her forearm at the same time. Although she had no numbness or tingling sensation, the simple acts of holding a book or a coffee cup, shaking hands, or turning a doorknob caused Christina intolerable pain. She stopped playing tennis, golf, and any other sports that might have caused the pain, and her doctor told her to take Tylenol or Advil, but when nothing helped diminish the pain, she decided to consult me.

In the course of performing a physical examination on Christina, I realized she was experiencing severe tenderness in both the lateral and medial parts of her elbow. The pain increased when I asked her to extend her wrist or flex it, and I concluded that Christina might have both tennis elbow (lateral epicondylitis) and golf elbow (medial epicondylitis), later determining that Christina has tennis elbow, which does not necessarily come from playing tennis, much as golf elbow does not necessarily come from playing golf.

SYMPTOMS, CAUSES, AND DIAGNOSIS

The painful symptoms that accompany these conditions have several root causes:

- Recreational sports, including fencing, a ground stroke in tennis, racquetball, or squash.

- Occupational tasks associated with painting, playing musical instruments, plumbing, raking, weaving, and the like.

It is the repetitive wrist extension and wrist flexing that can cause both tennis and golf elbow—the inflammation of the medial and lateral epicondyles. The diagnosis of both these conditions is routinely done by taking the person's history and giving a physical examination. X-rays are not necessary, although an MRI can occasionally be indicated to show any changes in the tendon at the site of its attachment to the bone.

TREATMENTS FOR BILATERAL ELBOW PAIN IN WESTERN MEDICINE

Noninvasive Treatments

Tennis and golf elbow can be treated nonsurgically or surgically. Nonsurgical treatments include the following.

Rest

Rest and cessation of any activity that may have caused the condition.

Ice Packs

Ice packs applied to the outside and inside parts of the elbow.

Medications

Ingestion of acetaminophen or other anti-inflammatory medications for pain relief.

Orthotics

Orthotics to diminish the symptoms. An elbow splint, the orthotic for this condition (see Figure 20.1), should be put tightly on the elbow in order to prevent it from stretching the lateral and medial epicondyle tendons.

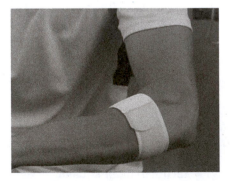

Figure 20.1

Physical Therapy

Physical therapy, using such methods as ultrasound and stretches. Stretches should be performed four times a day for a minute each to address tight structures in both parts of the forearm (see Figures 20.3 and 20.4). To prevent future problems, strengthening exercises are also implemented before allowing a return to full activity. These include wrist roll-ups, both up and down slowly to work both parts of the forearm. (See Figure 20.5.)

Invasive Treatments

Steroid Injections

Steroids, such as cortisone, are very effective anti-inflammatory medicines. If the physical therapy and other treatments failed, it might be

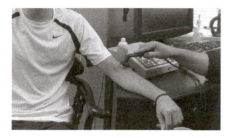

Figure 20.2

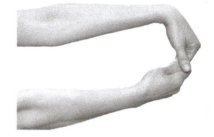

Figure 20.3

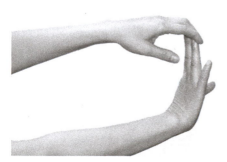

Figure 20.4

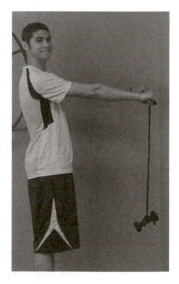

Figure 20.5

medically necessary to inject a steroid into your damaged muscle in order to relieve your symptoms.

Surgery

After 6 to 12 months of nonsurgical treatments without any improvement, surgery might be recommended. Most surgical procedures for tennis elbow involve removing diseased muscle and reattaching healthy muscle back to bone.

> *Open surgery.* The most common approach to tennis elbow repair is open surgery. This involves making an incision over the elbow.
>
> *Arthroscopic surgery.* Tennis elbow can also be repaired using tiny instruments and small incisions. Like open surgery, this is a same-day or outpatient procedure.

TREATMENTS FOR BILATERAL ELBOW PAIN IN TRADITIONAL CHINESE MEDICINE

Acupuncture

Acupuncture is very effective if started early and at the correct acupuncture points.

> *For lateral epicondylitis,* I use LI 10 Shou San Li, LI 11 Qu Chi, LI 12 Zhou Liao, and Arshi points.

The Arshi points should be selected in this manner. I feel the tendons of the lateral epicondyle touching the radial head and then insert the needles between the bone and tendon in order to separate them. Usually two to four Arshi points are picked up and then electrical stimulation should be applied with as high an intensity as is tolerable for about 25–30 minutes. (See Figures 20.6 and 20.7.)

> *For medial epicondylitis,* I pick up Heart 3 Xiao Hai and 3–4 Arshi points. The Arshi points will also be picked up to follow the tendon of the wrist flexors and to find the attachment of the tendon and the bone.

I vertically insert three or four needles along the tendon attachment with the bone and then start the use of electrical stimulation. As mentioned earlier, a high level of electrical stimulation should be applied for about 25–30 minutes. (See Figures 20.6 and 20.7 and Table 20.1.)

Table 20.1

	Points	Meridian/Number	Location	Conditions Helped
1	Shou San Li	LI 10	Between LI 5 and Li 11, 2 inch below LI 11	Abdominal pain, diarrhea, toothache, swelling of the cheek, motor impairment of the upper limbs, pain in the shoulder and back
2	Qu Chi	LI 11	*See* Table 14.1/Figure 14.4.	*See* Table 14.1.
3	Zhou Liao	LI 12	When the elbow is flexed, the point is superior to the lateral epicondyle of the humerus, about 1 inch superolateral to LI 11, on the medial border of the humerus.	Pain, numbness, and contracture of the elbow and arm
4	Xiao Hai	Heart 3	When the elbow is flexed into a right angle, the point is in the depression between the medial ends of the transverse crease of the wrist.	Chest pain, spasmodic pain of the elbow and arm, sudden loss of voice

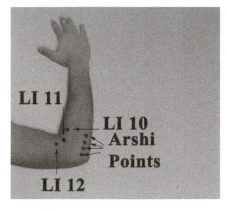

Figure 20.6

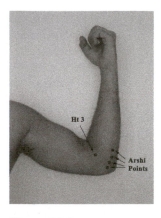

Figure 20.7

Follow-Up to Acupuncture

After the acupuncture points' stimulation, it is very important to follow up with an acupressure massage. This should be a friction massage that will attempt to detach the adhesion of the inflamed tendon to the bone and gradually loosen this attachment. This will greatly help diminish the pain and stiffness of both tennis and golf elbow.

CHRISTINA'S TREATMENT

In Christina's case, neither surgery nor steroid injections were necessary. She was, instead, treated for three weeks with a combination of acupuncture, acupressure, and massages, and during this time she was strongly advised not to play her violin. After three weeks, her tennis elbow was immensely improved, and she was taught to do her own massage and acupressure that would help keep her pain-free in the future.

TIPS FOR PEOPLE WITH BILATERAL ELBOW PAIN

- You should put ice on the tender points and then try to perform the friction massage for 15 minutes twice a day.
- Stop doing such sports as tennis or golf, as well as any other upper extremity activities. Depending on your condition, you should forgo these activities for at least one month or more.

TIPS FOR ACUPUNCTURE PRACTITIONERS

- The correct needle insertion involves inserting them between the bone and the tendons. This is to try and separate the adhesion between the inflamed tendon and bone.
- For the correct use of the friction massage, put your fingertips over the tendon's head at 90 degrees and perform the massage, in order to detach the adhesion between the inflamed tendon and bone.

21

Wrist Pain

Margaret, a 45-year-old pianist and professor in a New York school of music, spent a year preparing for a European concert, and was practicing for it much more than she normally does. A month before she was due to depart, she began experiencing a sharp pain in her left wrist, which became constant and severe. It originated near the base of her thumb and then gradually spread farther into her thumb and back into her forearm. When she played the piano, or tried to grasp an object, her wrist felt the sharp pain. She also felt some numbness on the back of the left thumb and index finger. Additionally, she found a fluid-filled cyst on her left wrist and had difficulty moving that wrist and thumb. Fearing she might have to cancel the European concert, she was extremely nervous and upset when she consulted me.

On examination, I found Margaret's left wrist to be a bit swollen and extremely tender, especially at the base of the thumb. At that point, she was unable to bend her wrist or grasp a book or a cup, I suspected that she had de Quervain tenosynovitis. As shown in Figure 21.1, I performed the Finkelstein test on her to determine the source of her pain. I had her hold her thumb in the palm of her hand and bend her wrist toward the little finger. This immediately exacerbated the pain, which confirmed my diagnosis of de Quervain tenosynovitis, an inflammation of the tendons on the side of the wrist at the base of the thumb.

SYMPTOMS, CAUSES, AND DIAGNOSIS

Dr. De Quervain was a Swiss surgeon who first identified this condition in 1895. There are two tendons—extensor pollicis brevis and abductor pollicis longus—which run side by side and pass through the wrist in the synovial sheath that contains them and allows them to exercise their function

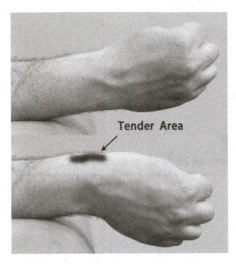

Figure 21.1

of moving the thumb away from the hand.

Some doctors think the cause of de Quervain tenosynovitis is unknown; others believe it is caused by repetitive exercise, such as Margaret's piano playing. The overuse of these two tendons can cause wrist pain, swelling, and even numbness, or a tingling sensation if the nerve is pinched. This second diagnosis also includes osteoarthritis at the base of the thumb.

TREATMENTS FOR WRIST PAIN IN WESTERN MEDICINE

Noninvasive Treatments

There are various ways of treating this condition nonsurgically.

Medications

Nonsteroidal anti-inflammatory drugs, such as ibuprofen, naproxen, or Aleve, can be given.

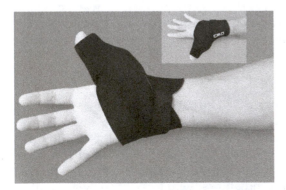

Figure 21.2

Immobilization

Natural treatments include immobilizing the thumb by using a spica splint. This fixes and immobilizes the thumb, promoting total rest and avoiding any thumb movements. (See Figure 21.2.)

Hot or Cold Treatments

Hot/cold treatment can be effective. Start with a heating pad on the affected area. This induces a lot of blood to flow to the affected thumb and wrist, which flushes away the inflammatory factors. Followed by ice packs, this serves to drive away the inflammatory fluids.

Invasive Treatment

Injections

Steroid injections are often extremely effective.

TREATMENTS FOR WRIST PAIN IN TRADITIONAL CHINESE MEDICINE

Acupuncture

There are three important points to utilize in acupuncture treatment for this condition.

The large intestine 4 He Gu serves to increase the endorphin secretion in the brain. It can synchronize with local points to decrease the pain and sensation in the brain.

The large intestine 5 Yang Xi and San Jiao 4 Yang Chi, LI 5 are the points located exactly between the tendons of extensor pollicis brevis and abductor pollicis longus. SJ 4 is adjacent to LI 5, which will help in the healing effects of LI 5. Heating and electrically stimulating the two needles can increase the amount of blood around the area and wash away the inflammation; the electrical stimulation will continually increase the energy flow to the area to decrease the feeling of pain.

The large intestine 11 Qu Chi is the point along

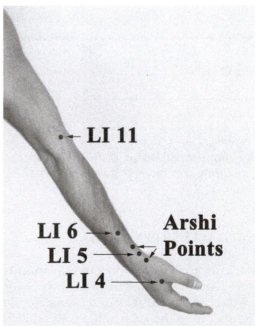

Figure 21.3

Table 21.1

	Points	Meridian/ Number	Location	Conditions Helped
1	He Gu	LI 4	See Table 13.1/ Figure 13.4.	See Table 13.1.
2	Yang Xi	LI 5	On the radial side of the wrist, when the thumb is tilted upward, it is in the depression between the tendons of m. extensor pollicis longus and brevis.	Headaches, redness, pain, and swelling of the eye, toothache, sore throat, pain in the wrist
3	Yang Chi	SJ 4	On the transverse crease of the dorsum of wrist, in the depression lateral to the tendon of m. extensor digitorum communis. See Figure 11.1.	Pain in the arm, shoulder, and wrist, malaria, deafness, thirst
4	Qu Chi	LI 11	See Figure 14.4/ Table 14.1.	See Table 14.1.

the same meridian of LI 5. LI 11 can assist in decreasing the pain by activating the energy from the distal meridian. (See Table 21.1 and Figure 21.3.)

MARGARET'S TREATMENT

Margaret received acupuncture treatments three times a week for four weeks and then came in twice a week for an additional six visits with the electrical stimulation and heated needle treatments. At the same time, she also wore the spica splint constantly and gave her wrist an ice massage immediately after her piano practice. Her pain was so improved that she was able to keep her concert date in Europe. She had a wonderfully successful tour and brought me back two CDs of her performance there.

TIPS FOR PEOPLE WITH WRIST PAIN

- The sooner treatment is commenced, the better chance you have of recovering. You should not wait to consult your doctor.
- Rest and immobilization are necessary. Many physicians think the condition is idiopathic (unknown), but my observation is that most likely it is the mechanical repetitions of the thumb that cause this condition.
- After acupuncture, heating, and electrical stimulation, it is best to apply ice to the wrist, which, in turn, helps decrease the inflammation.

TIPS FOR ACUPUNCTURE PRACTITIONERS

- In addition to the points listed in Table 21.1, you may add a few Arshi points along the insertional tendons of extensor pollicis brevis and abductor pollicis longus. For this it is crucial to know that the distal tendons are located in the lateral wrists, also called the snuff box.
- You need to recommend wearing the spica splint, which will immobilize the wrist and accelerate the healing process.

22

Carpal Tunnel Syndrome

Jessica is a 35-year-old computer programmer who, for the last 15 years, has worked roughly 10 hours a day on the computer. Two years ago she started to feel a numbness in her right hand with a tingling sensation along her thumb, index, and middle fingers that often occurs while holding a steering wheel, phone, newspaper, or upon awakening. She very often shook out her right hand to try and relieve symptoms, especially when the pain interfered with her sleep by waking her up. As the disorder progressed, the numb feeling became constant. Sometimes she also felt right wrist pain radiating up the arm to the shoulder, and down to the palm, especially at end of a long day spent typing. She had difficulty holding a book or a cup and very often dropped objects. She tried massaging her hand and wrist but felt no improvement, and at that point, she came to me for evaluation and treatment.

I performed a physical examination, and found that, while squeezing her right palm together and holding it for two minutes, she began to feel a numbness and a tingling sensation in her thumb, index, and middle fingers. The muscles of her right thumb and the side of her right palm were slightly atrophied, and the sensation was decreased. Suspecting that Jessica had carpal tunnel syndrome, I performed two tests.

1. *Tinel's sign.* I used my hammer to tap lightly on the middle line of the wrist, so Jessica would feel the sensation of tingling or pins and needles in the first three fingers.
2. *Phalen's maneuver.* I held Jessica's hand and flexed her wrist about 60–80 degrees and then waited for one minute, which caused her to feel numbness and tingling along the nerve (see Figures 22.1 and 22.2).

These tests confirmed for me that Jessica most likely had carpal tunnel syndrome, a condition that is often caused by the type of repetitive movement used in the computer work she did.

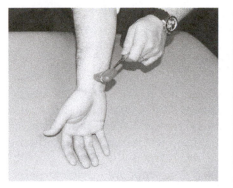

Figure 22.1

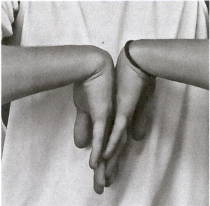

Figure 22.2

SYMPTOMS, CAUSES, AND DIAGNOSIS

The carpal tunnel is located at the midline of the palm adjacent to the wrist, and inside it lies the median nerve. This is a mixed nerve, meaning it has both sensory and motor functions. It sends out nerve signals to move your muscles and also provides feeling in your thumb, index finger, middle finger, and the middle-finger side of the ring finger. Pressure on the nerve can stem from anything that reduces the space for it in the carpal tunnel (see Figure 22.3).

There are several causes of carpal tunnel syndrome, but in most cases the cause is unknown.

Genetic predisposition. Many families have a tendency toward carpal tunnel syndrome. Where this complaint runs in the family, about 50 percent are women. It may be that their carpal tunnel is narrower than average.

Professionally related. Though there is some controversy over this, certain professions, such as data-entry technicians, secretaries, or construction workers, have higher chances of developing carpal tunnel syndrome. Repetitive flexing and extending

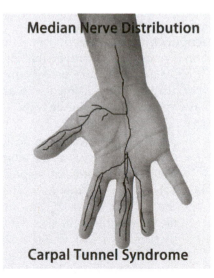

Median Nerve Distribution

Carpal Tunnel Syndrome

Figure 22.3

of the tendons in the hands and wrists, particularly when done forcefully and for prolonged periods without rest, can increase pressure within the carpal tunnel. Also, an injury to your wrist can cause swelling that exerts pressure on the median nerve.

Conditions such as hypothyroidism, multiple myeloma, pregnancy, rheumatoid arthritis, or trauma can compress the median nerve and cause the symptoms of carpal tunnel syndrome. If the condition is treated, or the pregnancy has come to term, then carpal tunnel syndrome will gradually disappear.

In diagnosing carpal tunnel syndrome, your symptoms are the most important factor. As mentioned earlier, if you have a numbness and tingling sensation in the thumb, index, middle finger, and half of the ring finger; if you wake up and shake your hand to try and relieve the pain and numbness in it; if you frequently drop an object, such as a book, a cup, or a pen, the diagnosis of carpal tunnel syndrome is suspected.

A physical examination can determine the condition. Sometimes tapping the front of the wrist can reproduce the tingling in the hand, and this is referred to as Tinel's sign of carpal tunnel syndrome. Symptoms can also at times be reproduced when the examiner bends the wrist forward, and this is referred to as Phalen's maneuver.

Nerve conduction velocity test (NCV) and electromyogram (EMG) are two electrophysiological tests that are considered the gold standard for diagnosing carpal tunnel syndrome. Usually a physical examination coupled with complaints about your condition is sufficient to make an accurate diagnosis. But the final diagnosis depends on the electrophysiological testing that will not only tell you the diagnosis but also the types of treatment and the prognosis—whether your condition needs physical therapy, acupuncture, brace, steroid injection, or surgery; or whether your condition is reversible, nonreversible, or similar.

NCV and EMG are usually performed by physiatrists, doctors who specialize in physical medicine and rehabilitation, or neurologists who have special training in the tests.

- *The NCV test* involves mild to moderate electrical stimulation of the median nerves at the elbows and wrists of both sides. A computer will record the responses of the nerves and compare the velocity, amplitude, and latency. By comparing the results with the normal standard, and also comparing the left-side median nerve with the right side, your doctor can identify whether or not there is any injury to the median nerves.
- *The EMG test* inserts a very fine needle into your muscles at the palm, arm, and neck. The needle contains a microscopic electrode, which

picks up both normal and abnormal electrical signals given off by a muscle. If there is nerve damage, the muscles supplied by the nerve will send out abnormal signals. Because the median nerve originates from the cervical spine on the neck and goes through the entire arm and lateral palm, some muscles will be examined with the needles. The test usually will take about 30 minutes to an hour, depending on how severe your condition and how extensive a study your physician chooses to do. You may feel mild discomfort with the test, but 99.9 percent of my patients easily take the test I perform.

Blood tests may be done to identify any medical conditions associated with carpal tunnel syndrome. They include complete blood counts, blood sugar and protein analysis, and thyroid hormone levels.

X-ray tests of the wrist and hand might also be helpful to identify abnormalities of the bones and joints of the wrist.

TREATMENTS FOR CARPAL TUNNEL SYNDROME IN WESTERN MEDICINE

Noninvasive Treatments

There are three types of carpal tunnel syndrome: mild, moderate, and severe, and how these are determined and treated depends on their symptoms and the electrophysiological testing.

Braces/Splints

For mild and moderate cases, immobilizing braces are recommended. A wrist splint can help limit numbness by preventing wrist flexing, which might compress the median nerve. You should wear a night splint, usually called a cock-up splint, and the wrist should be extended out. (See Figure 22.4.) Worn overnight for 7–8 hours, it will rest the nerves, and in the morning you will feel relieved and the symptoms will gradually improve.

Physical Therapy

Stretching is very important to improve mobility in the wrist and get rid of any restrictions and inflammation in the carpal tunnel,

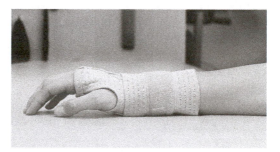

Figure 22.4

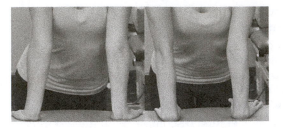

Figure 22.5

where the tendons of the wrist and the median nerve pass through. To perform this stretch, pull the fingers and thumb back with your palm facing away from the body. This stretch for the wrist can be done by placing your hand on a wall or a table. (See Figure 22.5.) A strong but comfortable stretch should be performed four times a day and held one minute.

The American Academy of Orthopedic Surgeons recommends ultrasound as a treatment option to assist with short- and medium-term benefits of carpal tunnel.

Even with all the treatment approaches listed, if the underlying problems, such as improper stresses on the hands while at work, are not corrected, the carpal tunnel problem will resurface. Physical therapists play an important part in educating you on proper ergonomics, and they sometimes even visit work sites to properly set up office spaces and ensure proper arm and wrist position.

Medications

Western medicine also uses nonsteroid anti-inflammatory drugs, such as Aleve and naproxen, or even some steroid drugs taken orally.

Invasive Treatments

Steroid Injections

Localized steroid injections can be used for mild and moderate forms of this syndrome and are very effective for temporary relief. However, these injections are not recommended for severe carpal tunnel syndrome (see Figure 22.6).

Surgery

For severe carpal tunnel syndrome, surgery is the best option. The two major types are open hand surgery and endoscopic surgery.

In open hand surgery, your surgeon performs carpal tunnel release by cutting the tissue that holds joints together (the carpal ligament) to relieve the pressure on your median nerve. You'll have local or regional anesthesia and will usually go home soon after your surgery. This procedure usually results in significant improvement in your symptoms, but you still may experience some residual numbness, pain, or weakness.

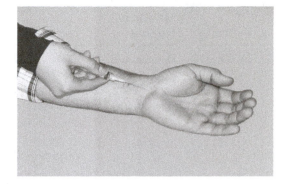

Figure 22.6

In endoscopic surgery, your surgeon performs carpal tunnel release through one or two small incisions in your hand or wrist, using a device with a tiny camera attached to it (an endoscope) to see inside the carpal tunnel.

TREATMENTS FOR CARPAL TUNNEL SYNDROME IN TRADITIONAL CHINESE MEDICINE

Acupuncture

Acupuncture is very effective for the mild to moderate forms of this syndrome. The points used are PC 7 Da Ling and PC 6 Nei Guan. After inserting the needles at these two points, it is usually effective to introduce electrical stimulation in the direction of the fingertip. You should feel the needle sensation radiating to the tips of the fingers; sometimes it swells and feels sore as you experience the electrical shock to the fingertip.

This treatment is most effective when it is performed three times a week for a month, and a cock-up splint (see Figure 22.4) is also worn at night while sleeping. Many people get excellent results from the combination of these two treatments (see Table 22.1 and Figure 22.7).

JESSICA'S TREATMENT

Jessica underwent my treatment for a total of 12 visits. In addition to the acupuncture, she used a cock-up splint at night and rested her hand by not typing for one month. Gradually, as her symptoms diminished, she felt much less of the numbness and tingling sensation, and her hands recovered their strength as well.

Table 22.1

	Points	Meridian/Number	Location	Conditions Helped
1	Da Ling	Pericardium 7	In the middle of the transverse crease of the wrist, between the tendons of palmaris longus and flexor carpi radialis	Cardiac pain, palpitations, stomach ache, vomiting, mental disorders, epilepsy, stuffy chest pain, convulsions, insomnia, irritability, foul breath, pain in the elbow, arm and hand
2	Nei Guan	Pericardium 6	2 inches above the transverse crease of the wrist, between the tendons of palmaris longus and flexor radialis	Cardiac pain, palpitations, stuffy chest, abdominal pain, stomach ache, nausea, vomiting, hiccups, mental disorders, epilepsy, insomnia, febrile diseases, irritability, malaria, contracture and pain of the elbow, arm, and hand
3	Qu Ze	Pericardium 3	On the transverse cubital crease, at the ulnar side of the tendon of biceps brachii	Cardiac pain, palpitations, febrile diseases, irritability, stomach ache, vomiting, pain in the elbow, arm, and hand, tremors of the hand and arm

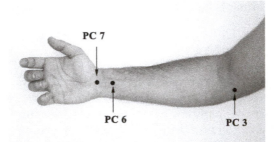

Figure 22.7

TIPS FOR PEOPLE WITH CARPAL TUNNEL SYNDROME

- Be sure you get an accurate diagnosis. Some people feel numbness in their hands and fingers, but don't have carpal tunnel syndrome. These conditions could also be symptomatic of arthritis, so if the diagnosis is incorrect, the treatments listed here won't help you.
- Try to wear the cock-up splint as much as possible, not just at night, but also while driving or doing daily chores. This will help give the nerve and carpal tunnel a rest and help speed recovery.

TIPS FOR ACUPUNCTURE PRACTITIONERS

- A clear diagnosis is necessary. Some patients feel numbness and tingling in their fingers and hands without having carpal tunnel syndrome. These sensations might be due to rheumatoid arthritis, osteoarthritis, or other causes, and if the diagnosis is not correct, the acupuncture and a cock-up splint cannot help.
- The insertion of the acupuncture needles in the two points, PC 7 and PC 6, should not be too deep, about 1/3 inch. The electrical stimulation should be as strong as possible while still being tolerable so it will bring enough energy to flow through the carpal tunnel and decrease the swelling of the hand.
- I usually encourage the patient to wear the cock-up splint not only at night but as much as is practicable during the day, while driving or doing daily chores. This will greatly improve the patient's resting the median nerve and the carpal tunnel.

23

Ulnar Nerve Entrapment

Derek is a 43-year-old man who likes to cycle cross country. He has regularly biked 100 miles a week for over 10 years. On weekends he will get up early in the morning and participate in a very intensive bike ride. Some months back, he started to feel that his hands were weak and tender, as well as numb, and he felt coldness and a tingling sensation on the fourth and fifth fingers of both hands. He sometimes had difficulty typing and had to shake his hands to rid himself of the numbness after waking up. He visited his primary care physician, was given Advil for his pain, and told that after a few weeks the pain and numbness might go away. However, he still felt it and it was getting worse, so he came to me for evaluation and treatment.

Because the ulnar nerve goes to the fourth and fifth fingers, Derek's symptoms made me think it was ulnar nerve entrapment, also called Guyon's canal syndrome, a common nerve compression affecting the ulnar nerve as it passes through a tunnel in the wrist called Guyon's canal. This problem is similar to carpal tunnel syndrome but involves a completely different nerve. By physical examination, Derek showed a weakness when trying to make a full fist, and even more weakness when he went to spread out his five fingers.

SYMPTOMS, CAUSES, AND DIAGNOSIS

The ulnar nerve is one of the three main nerves in the arm. It is located underneath the shoulder, and runs along the arm to the little and ring fingers. In this pathway, there are a few locations where the ulnar nerve can be easily trapped, as indicated in Figure 23.1.

The ulnar nerve functions to give sensation to the little finger and the half of the ring finger that is near the little finger. It also controls most of the little muscles in the hand that help with fine movements, and some of the bigger muscles in the forearm that help to make a strong grip.

As the ulnar nerve travels from under the collarbone and along the inside of the upper arm, it passes through the cubital tunnel of tissue behind the inside of the elbow. You can feel the sensation commonly called the funny bone when you place your elbow on the desk to answer your phone, or when you lie on your stomach holding your arm face down.

Below the elbow, the nerve travels under muscles on the inside of the arm and into the hand on the side of the palm with the little finger. As the nerve enters the hand, it travels through another tunnel called Guyon's canal. The most common injury to this area results from riding a bicycle for a long time, as in Derek's case (see Figures 23.1 to 23.3).

The ulnar nerve originates from the neck. If you bend your neck to the side often, it is easy to pinch the nerve on the neck, as shown in Figures 23.4 to 23.6.

Symptoms of ulnar nerve entrapment can vary from a mild, transient pins-and-needles sensation in the ring and small fingers to a frozen clawing of these digits and severe intrinsic muscle atrophy. The person may report severe pain at the elbow or wrist, with radiation into the hand or up into the shoulder and neck, and may experience difficulty opening jars, spreading out the hand and fingers, or turning doorknobs. This can be accompanied by fatigue or weakness after repetitive hand motions, such as typing or

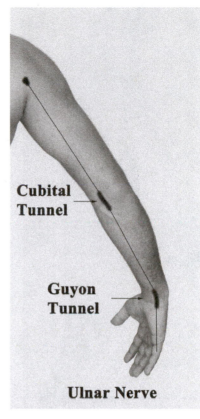

Figure 23.1

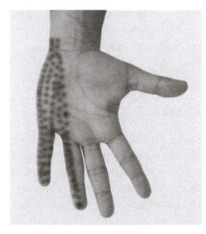

Figure 23.2

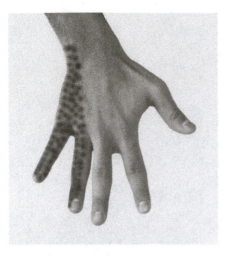

Figure 23.3

Figure 23.4

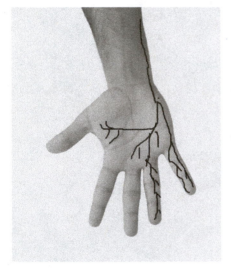

Figure 23.5

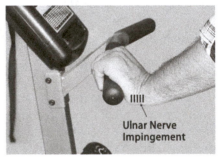

Ulnar Nerve
Impingement

Figure 23.6

sorting mail. Increasing numbness and other abnormal sensations, paresthesias such as prickling or tingling, may be noticed throughout the day.

Ulnar neuropathy can be caused by nerve damage, which can result from inflammation or compression along the pathway of the ulnar nerve in the following instances.

- Bicycle riding
- Blunt injuries with or without fracture

- Blunt trauma
- Compression at work, sleep, or during general anesthesia
- Damage at or near the elbow
- Deformities, including rheumatoid arthritis or fracture of elbow bones
- Ganglionic cysts
- Hemophilia, leading to hematomas
- Malnutrition leading to muscle atrophy and loss of fatty protection in the elbow and other joints
- Metabolic syndrome (common with diabetes)
- Tumors
- Ulnar neuropathy in Guyon's canal
- Unknown (idiopathic)
- Venipuncture

A proper diagnosis of ulnar nerve entrapment depends on an experienced physician who does the following:

- Takes a clear medical history, asking you details, including when, where, and how, the symptoms started.
- Performs a comprehensive medical examination that includes inspection of any muscle atrophy, feeling the tender area, tests for range of motion, sensitivity, and special muscle strength.
- Does electrodiagnostic studies (EMG) to study nerve conduction in your hands and wrists, which is a gold standard for the final diagnosis of ulnar neuropathy.

TREATMENTS FOR ULNAR NERVE ENTRAPMENT IN WESTERN MEDICINE

Noninvasive Treatments

The choice of treatment depends on the severity of your symptoms. For mild to moderate ulnar neuropathy, such treatments as physical or occupational therapy, nonsteroidal anti-inflammatory medicine, and splints are recommended.

Physical Therapy

Physical therapy can stretch, strengthen, and remove adhesions in the ligaments and tendons in the hands and elbows.

The ulnar nerve gliding maneuver (see Figure 23.7), where the hand is upside down with the fingers around the eye, can help unblock the

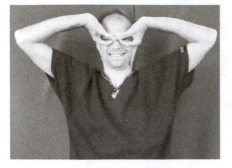

Figure 23.7

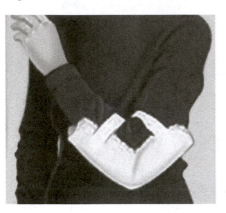

Figure 23.8

entrapment. Repeat this three times, holding for 20 seconds each time.

Medications

The daily use of nonsteroidal anti-inflammatory drugs, such as aspirin, ibuprofen, and other non-prescription pain relievers, can help reduce pain and inflammation.

Splints

Wearing splints can help immobilize and protect the elbow and wrist (see Figure 23.8).

Invasive Treatment

Surgery

For severe cases, and after conservative treatments have been tried, the following methods are considered:

At the elbow. Your surgeon will make an incision at the elbow and perform a nerve decompression. Or your surgeon may choose to move the nerve to the inner part of the arm so it is in a more direct position.

At the wrist. If the compression is at the wrist, the incision is made there and the nerve decompression is performed.

TREATMENTS FOR ULNAR NERVE ENTRAPMENT IN TRADITIONAL CHINESE MEDICINE

Acupuncture

The most commonly used points for this condition are SI 4 Wan Gu, SI 5 Yang Gu, SI 6 Yang Lao, SI 7 Zhi Zheng, and SI 8 Xiao Hai (see Table 23.1 and Figure 23.9).

Table 23.1

	Points	Meridian/ Number	Location	Conditions Helped
1	Wan Gu	SI 4	On the ulnar side of the palm, in the depression between the base of the 5th metacarpal bone and the triquetral bone	Febrile diseases with inability to sweat normally, headaches, rigidity of the neck, contracture of the fingers, pain in the wrist, jaundice
2	Yang Gu	SI 5	At the ulnar end of the transverse crease on the dorsal aspect of the wrist, in the depression between the styloid process of the ulnar and the triquetral bone	Swelling of the neck and the region under the jaw, pain in the hand and wrist, febrile diseases
3	Yang Lao	SI 6	Dorsal to the head of the ulna. When the palm faces the chest, the point is in the bony cleft on the radial side of the styloid process of the ulna.	Blurring of vision, pain in the shoulder, elbow, and arm
4	Zhi Zheng	SI 7	On the line joining SI 5 Yang Gu and SI 8 Xiao Hai, 5 inch above Yang Gu	Neck rigidity, headaches, dizziness, spasmodic pain in the elbow and fingers, febrile diseases, mania
5	Xiao Hai	SI 8	When the elbow is flexed, the point is located in the depression between the olecranon of the ulna and the medial epicondyle of the humerus.	Headaches, swelling in the cheek, pain in the shoulder, arm, and elbow, epilepsy

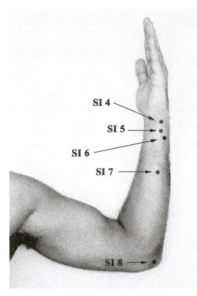

Figure 23.9

DEREK'S TREATMENT

Derek underwent treatment with me three times a week for four weeks. I mainly selected SI4 and SI8, which are major blockage locations of the ulnar nerve. After the needles were first inserted, Derek felt a sharp sensation, and following that he felt some warmth traveling from the wrist to the elbow. His numbness and tingling decreased after three or four treatments, and after 10 visits, he felt completely cured, but to make sure, I continued treatments for another two sessions.

TIPS FOR PEOPLE WITH ULNAR NERVE ENTRAPMENT

- Avoid pressing down on your elbow or wrist during sports or work.
- If the sensation of numbness and tingling in the ring and little fingers is on and off for a short period, that is, it is temporary, it will usually disappear without treatment. However, if you constantly press on your elbow and wrist, you may develop permanent damage.

TIPS FOR ACUPUNCTURE PRACTITIONERS

- Make a clear diagnosis, and make sure to check the causes of the ulnar neuropathy. Acupuncture may not affect the causes of this condition.
- Early treatment will help relieve the problem, but acupuncture may only help with the symptoms. For permanent relief, patients need to change their ways of practicing sports or working.

24

Dupuytren's Contracture

Luke, a 72-year-old man who was born in Norway, reported that about a year ago he noticed a small lump growing along the fourth finger of his right hand that continued to the area where his palm and fourth finger meet. In the beginning, his finger felt only slightly tender; but six months later, the finger had gradually contracted and he experienced difficulty extending the finger at the metacarpal phalangeal, proximal interphalangeal, and distal interphalangeal finger joints. Though he did not experience much pain, he did notice there was a cord of tissue under the skin of his palm that prevented him from extending his fourth finger and greatly interfered with his hand function and movement. This situation continued to develop over a year, at which point he went to his primary care physician who did not understand what was wrong with Luke's hand. Luke was then referred to me.

In examining Luke's hand, I too noticed a cordlike tissue that had formed along his fourth finger and had caused it to bend unnaturally toward his palm. There did not seem to be much tenderness in the area, but Luke had difficulty extending his fourth finger and coordinating it with his other fingers. He had tried massage, ultrasound, and physical therapy, including stretching exercises for the hand, but none of it helped and his symptoms were gradually getting worse, leading me to believe he had a condition known as Dupuytren's contracture.

SYMPTOMS, CAUSES, AND DIAGNOSIS

Dupuytren's contracture is a very specific condition. It often affects people of Scandinavian or Northern European descent and has been called the *Viking Disease,* though it has also been found in Spain and the Far East.

Its primary characteristics include the following:

- People who are older than 40 are the ones most likely to develop the condition. For anyone older than 40, the disease is more common in men than in women. By age 80, however, gender is not an important factor.
- It is often a condition that is passed down through families.
- It usually happens in the fourth and fifth fingers; the thumb and index fingers are almost always spared.
- Some may contract Dupuytren's after developing certain conditions, such as alcoholism, diabetes, epilepsy, liver disease, or trauma.

Although Dupuytren's contracture is poorly understood, many physicians and research scientists think it is caused by fibroblast proliferation and collagen deposits.

It is thought there are three stages of Dupuytren's contracture.

The proliferation stage, which is characterized by the development of nodules. Many of the nodules may be located or felt at the far end of the palm's crease.

The active stage, in which the cord begins to form near the nodule.

The residual stage, in which tendonlike cords are visible and the contraction between the palm and fingers becomes obvious.

TREATMENTS FOR DUPUYTREN'S CONTRACTURE IN WESTERN MEDICINE

Noninvasive Treatments

It is not usually necessary to treat this condition. However, if you develop the later stage of this condition, up to the point where your finger function becomes restricted, it may be necessary to seek medical treatment.

Collagenase Injections

This treatment, currently in phase three of FDA approval, utilizes an injection of collagenase along the contracted cords. A small dosage of collagenase is best to dissolve or soften the cords.

X-Rays

Low-energy X-rays can also soften or reduce the contraction of the cords.

Physical Therapy

Warming up the area is important, first with heat, then ultrasound. Manual work on the hand can help remove restrictions, and should be followed by stretches to regain more motion.

Invasive Treatment

Surgery

Surgery for this condition consists of opening the skin over the affected cords and removing the fibrous tissue. This procedure is not curative, however, and cannot prevent the affected wrist and palm areas from developing Dupuytren's disease again at a later date.

After the surgery, you will most likely need further surgery to clean out the remainder of the cord in your fingers. Also be advised that the surgery comes with a risk of injury to the nerves and surrounding connective tissues.

TREATMENTS FOR DUPUYTREN'S CONTRACTURE IN TRADITIONAL CHINESE MEDICINE

Acupuncture

Acupuncture is a minimally invasive technique. For this condition, the needles are inserted locally along the cords, and electrical stimulation is then added to the highest degree that can be tolerated. It lasts 25–30 minutes, and you are allowed to adjust the stimulation level yourself. This treatment is followed by five minutes of ultrasound to soften the cord. Finally, there is a massage and some stretching exercises, all of which together serve to decrease the rigidity of the cord. (See Table 24.1 and Figure 24.1.)

Table 24.1

	Points	Meridian/ Number	Location	Conditions Helped
1	He Gu	LI 4	*See* Figure 13.4/ Table 13.1.	*See* Table 13.1.
2	Qu Chi	LI 11	*See* Figure 14.4/ Table 14.1.	*See* Table 14.1.
3	Arshi		These are nonspecific points, and needles should be inserted along the shortened tendon as Figure 24.1.	

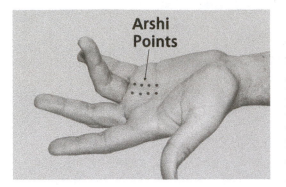

Arshi Points

Figure 24.1

LUKE'S TREATMENT

Luke underwent the combination of treatments discussed earlier 15 times. He was also told to soak his hand in very hot water every morning for 15–20 minutes, and to massage and stretch his fourth finger. He repeated these same stretches after acupuncture treatments in my office. After 15 visits, his condition was completely resolved. This treatment routine was also successfully tried in France in 1983, with similar positive results.

ADDITIONAL TREATMENTS FOR DUPUYTREN'S CONTRACTURE

I have treated more than 30 cases of Dupuytren's contracture and have found that the earlier the treatment, the better the results. For example, I treated a young, 25-year-old man who had a family history of Dupuytren's that had passed on to him. He had developed a nodule in his right hand at the meeting point of the fourth finger and palm. Because he consulted me at the earliest stage of his condition, I was able to cure him in only six or seven visits. If treatment is begun at a very late stage, acupuncture may not be a successful therapy.

TIPS FOR PEOPLE WITH DUPUYTREN'S CONTRACTURE

- Your cooperation in the treatment procedures is very important. This includes soaking your hands in hot water for 15–20 minutes every morning and doing stretching exercises on the affected finger.
- The results will be even better if you self-treat at home by massaging Chinese herbal massage cream or oil—red flower is good—into the affected area.

TIPS FOR ACUPUNCTURE PRACTITIONERS

- In treating Dupuytren's contracture, the needle should be inserted not only into the surface of the cord but also into the surrounding areas of the cords, and sometimes even beneath the cord. Adding electrical stimulation will maximize the treatment results.

- The patient's cooperation is a very important part of the treatment. You should tell the patient to soak his or her hands in hot water for 15–20 minutes each morning and do stretching exercises on the affected finger.
- The results will be even better if coupled with massages in the clinic and at home with Chinese herbal massage cream/oil, such as red flower. If the patient is assiduous in self-treatments and office visits, then surgery and its potentially negative side effects (possible nerve or vein injuries) can be avoided for early and mid-stage cases.

25

Hand Arthritis

Catherine is a 62-year-old woman who has had wrist pain for the past 10 years, and her pain had intensified significantly during the two months prior to her consulting me. She felt pain at the base of her right thumb, and the condition worsened in the morning because it was accompanied by stiffness, swelling, and, if pressed, tenderness. She also noticed redness and warmth in the area. Sometimes, the pain interfered with her daily activities, and she found it difficult to grasp everyday objects, such as books and cups.

My physical exam noted a slight to moderate deformity at the base of the right thumb and around the wrist, with severe tenderness at the thumb's base. Catherine's left thumb was also tender and slightly deformed. The range of motion for this thumb had decreased significantly, and the joint was very stiff and sensitive to touch or pressure.

I performed the Finkelstein test, but the results came back negative (the Finkelstein test evaluates the inflammation-associated pain of tendons on the lateral wrist). Jessica did not feel pain in the tendon during this test, but when I ordered an X-ray to examine the space between the joint and the scaphoid bone (situated between the hand and forearm on the thumb side of the wrist—also called the lateral, or radial, side), the results showed that the radius was very narrow and that the joint and the scaphoid were nearly bone on bone. I also noted the presence of a bone spur. The X-ray showed a slight dislocation of the joints at the base of the thumb, and I concluded that Catherine had obvious osteoarthritis on her right thumb.

SYMPTOMS, CAUSES, AND DIAGNOSIS

Hand osteoarthritis should be differentiated from two other conditions.

De Quervain tenosynovitis. As described previously, this is tendon inflammation, and in this case, the Finkelstein test would be positive (the Finkelstein test comes back negative if the problem is osteoarthritis).

Rheumatoid arthritis. This is a systemic condition that can affect the whole body and multiple joints. The symptoms are usually experienced symmetrically on both sides of the body. Rheumatoid arthritis causes deformity and instability. The inflammation always spreads to the tendons and the synovial tissue. This condition is confirmed via the existence of rheumatoid factors found through a blood test.

Although the cause of osteoarthritis is unknown, many doctors think it is due to a loss of cartilage. This may be due to disease or trauma, or it may be genetic. Children of people with this condition have a higher predisposition to develop it, and women are also more susceptible to osteoarthritis. Age, too, is often a factor.

A diagnosis of osteoarthritis is usually made by clinical examination and X-rays. It is not necessary to perform a CT, bone scan, arthroscopy.

TREATMENTS FOR HAND ARTHRITIS IN WESTERN MEDICINE

Noninvasive Treatments

Medications and Supplements

Anti-inflammatory medications, such as Tylenol and Advil, prescription drugs, such as Celebrex, and glucosamine-chondroitin supplements, can be taken to alleviate the pain. Though there is no definite evidence that glucosamine treats hand osteoarthritis, many of my patients use it to good effect.

Splinting

Splinting can help support the affected joints, decrease the pain, and ease the stress.

Physical Therapy

This will help improve pain-free range of motion through warming up the wrist; manual techniques, such as shown in Figure 25.1, upper arm bicycle, and Figure 25.2, twisting the clay, which will improve the flexibilities

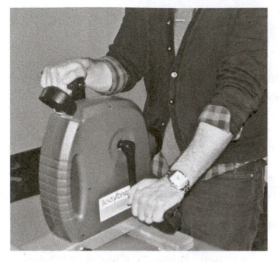

Figure 25.1

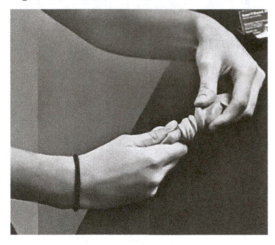

Figure 25.2

at each joint. These are followed by stretches and functional activities, such as turning a key to the left and right, and practicing key turns with putty.

Invasive Treatments

Injections

The most common injection is 1–2 percent lidocaine mixed with steroids. This can provide pain relief from a few weeks up to many months but can be repeated only a limited number of times because of its many potential side effects, such as dependency, joint weakness, infection, and lightening of the skin.

Surgery

If needed, several surgical procedures can be helpful.

- Thumb-base fusion utilizing a plate and screws.
- Joint replacement using a joint prosthesis.

TREATMENTS FOR HAND ARTHRITIS IN TRADITIONAL CHINESE MEDICINE

Acupuncture

There is a lot of evidence that acupuncture can decrease the pain of osteoarthritis. The needles are inserted into both sides of the joint line, and

Table 25.1

	Points	Meridian/ Number	Location	Conditions Helped
1	He Gu	LI 4	*See* Figure 23.4/Table 23.1.	*See* Table 23.1.
2	Qu Chi	LI 11	*See* Figure 24.4/Table 24.1.	*See* Table 24.1.
3	Arshi		*See* Figure 25.3.	

electrical stimulation and heat are applied as strongly as the patient can take, for 25 to 30 minutes.

Needles are then inserted head to head along the joint lines, and into the Arshi points He Gu LI 4 and Quchi LI 11. This acupuncture treatment is able to decrease the pain, but it will not correct any deformity or slow the progression of the osteoarthritis (see Table 25.1 and Figure 25.3).

CATHERINE'S TREATMENT

I treated Catherine for about 15 sessions. I chose the points described earlier and added electrical stimulation at the Arshi points. In the meantime, she was asked to do the previously

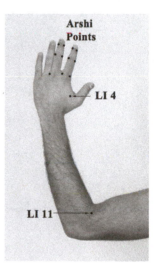

Figure 25.3

mentioned range-of-motion exercises with the joints of each hand twice a day, for 30 minutes each time. Catherine also was instructed to use a heating pad on both hands for 15 minutes and follow this with a cold pad. After a total of 15 sessions, she felt significant improvement.

TIPS FOR PEOPLE WITH HAND ARTHRITIS

- My personal experience has been that early treatment is far better than late treatment.
- You should soak your hands in hot water for 10 minutes each morning, massage each of the joints in your hand, and perform range-of-motion exercises for 10 minutes every day. By doing so, you will smooth the finger joints and relax the muscles in your hands.

TIPS FOR ACUPUNCTURE PRACTITIONERS

- If your patients do not show signs of acute inflammation, I would encourage you to add moxa to the needles for 8–10 minutes. You will get great effects if you use moxa to treat non-acutely inflamed hands.
- Electrical stimulation of the acupuncture needles, as well as heat, will go far to help relieve the symptoms and decrease the pain. The combination of acupuncture, physical therapy for improving range of motion, and stretching to increase joint mobility will significantly enhance joint function and is much more effective than any one treatment alone.

26

Trigger Finger

Madeline, a 60-year-old woman who works as a housekeeper, had been experiencing pain in the area of her right first finger joint near the palm (right metacarpophalangeal—MCP—joint) for about four months. As a housekeeper, she spent a lot of her time cleaning houses and was constantly opening and closing her hand at the joint of her right index finger, the exact point where she experienced the pain, tenderness, and redness. She ignored the condition for a month, but the pain became worse and she had difficulty extending the index finger. She could also feel her knuckles keeping her finger from sliding in and out, and her finger would sometimes get locked in a bent condition.

Upon examining Madeline, I discovered that she could bend the knuckle located at the base of the right index finger, but she had difficulty extending her index finger. When I forced the extension of this finger, the manipulation did succeed, but she felt extreme pain. She reported that in the mornings she could not move the finger at all until she had immersed it in hot water for 10 minutes.

Madeline has a condition known as trigger finger, which is the snapping of the digits when the hand is opened or closed.

SYMPTOMS, CAUSES, AND DIAGNOSIS

Trigger finger was first noted in soldiers who could not fire their weapons, due to inflammation of the right index finger caused by its repeated use. This condition, also called stenosing tenosynovitis, involves the hand's pulley and tendon system that governs the bending of the fingers. The pulley at the base of the finger becomes too thick, constricting the tendons and making it difficult for the finger to move freely through the pulley. Sometimes the tendon develops a knot or swelling at the base of the index finger. Trigger finger is different from Dupuytren's contracture, which causes the thickening and shortening of the connective tissue in the palm of the hand. Trigger finger, on the other hand, is characterized by inflammation of the pulley system in the finger that prevents the tendon from freely moving in and out of this system, with the result that the index finger is unable to flex or extend freely.

Trigger finger usually affects more men than women. It most commonly affects the index finger, or occasionally the thumb, and starts with discomfort felt at the base of the finger or thumb where they join the palm. The area often feels tender when pressure is applied, and a nodule may sometimes be found in this area. The person often thinks there is a problem with the middle or top knuckle of the digit after a nodule is found.

Risk Factors for Trigger Finger

- Repetitive grinding and gripping of the knuckles, such as repetitive use of power tools or musical instruments (especially bows for violins or cellos), for an extended period is a major risk for trigger finger.
- Some medical conditions, such as amyloidosis, diabetes, hypothyroidism, rheumatoid arthritis, or tuberculosis, leave people more prone to developing trigger finger.

TREATMENTS FOR TRIGGER FINGER IN WESTERN MEDICINE

Noninvasive Treatments

Rest

I always strongly advise my patients to rest the affected finger, with no gripping and no repetitive opening and closing of the hand.

Splinting

A splint can help keep the finger in the extended position, which rests the joint and decreases the inflammation. A brace may have to be worn for as long as six weeks.

Soaking and Massage

The patient is instructed to immerse the affected finger in hot water every morning for 15–20 minutes and then gently massage it and put ice on the finger for 10 min to help relieve the pain and soften the nodule.

Medications

Anti-inflammatory medications, such as ibuprofen, Advil, or Motrin, can decrease the swelling and inflammation of the trigger finger.

Invasive Treatments

Steroid Injections

Injections of steroids near or into the tendon sheaths usually reduce the inflammation of the cyst dramatically. This treatment is extremely effective.

Surgery

If none of the previously mentioned treatments are successful, it will be necessary to find a hand surgeon to perform a surgical release of the tendon.

TREATMENTS FOR TRIGGER FINGER IN TRADITIONAL CHINESE MEDICINE

Acupuncture

Acupuncture is also an effective treatment for trigger finger. Needles should be inserted directly along the nodule (the Arshi point). Electrical stimulation should be applied and ultrasound employed. Acupuncture needles with electrical stimulation that are inserted into the nodule for 30 minutes soften the hardened tissue at the trigger-finger joints.

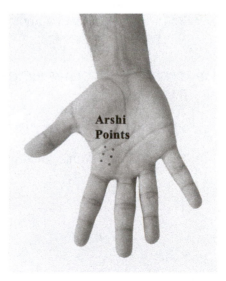

The ultrasound that follows can increase the blood flow around the nodule, and these three treatments, used together, can greatly decrease the inflammation of the nodule to such a degree that the person may not need any other treatment (see Table 26.1 and Figure 26.1).

Figure 26.1

Table 26.1

	Points	Meridian/Number	Location	Conditions Helped
1	He Gu	LI 4	*See* Figure 23.4/ Table 23.1.	*See* Table 23.1.
2	Qu Chi	LI 11	*See* Figure 24.4/ Table 24.1.	*See* Table 24.1.
3	Arshi		Needles are inserted along the tender nonspecific points called Arshi points. *See* Figure 26.1.	

MADELINE'S TREATMENT

Madeline underwent acupuncture and other treatments in traditional Chinese medicine for 10 visits. Her condition was so greatly improved that she experienced no more pain and was able to return to work.

TIPS FOR PEOPLE WITH TRIGGER FINGER

- My experience with trigger finger shows that it is most important for you to rest.
- You must also take care not to do any repetitive gripping during this period.

TIPS FOR ACUPUNCTURE PRACTITIONERS

- Early treatment with acupuncture, electrical stimulation, and ultrasound can be used effectively for mild to moderate trigger finger.
- Surgery, if called for, should be utilized only as a last resort.

27

Acute Low Back Sprain

Frank, a 35-year-old man, experienced sudden-onset low back pain for two days. He was moving a large piece of furniture for his girlfriend when he suddenly felt a pain in his lower back. It was constant and made it impossible for him to move his back. It was so severe, in fact, that it caused his entire back to spasm. The pain occurred from his lower back down to his buttocks, and though it did not radiate down his legs, or cause tingling or numbness, it became extremely difficult for him to put on his socks and pants. He did not experience any urinary incontinence or bowel or bladder abnormalities.

Frank's girlfriend took him to the emergency room, where he underwent an MRI that came back negative, showing he did not have a herniated disc. He also had an X-ray, which did not reveal a fracture. He was given pain medication and sent home, with instructions for two days of bed rest, during which time he had massages and heating pads that did not help him. When the pain had not abated after two days, and Frank could not sleep in his bed (he had to lie on the floor, instead) or go to work, he decided to come to me for a consultation.

My examination showed that Frank could only move his back forward about 30 degrees and could not bend backward or extend his back. When I touched his back, the entire back muscle went into spasm, and his cervical, thoracic, and lumbar spine areas were slightly twisted. Using a manual muscle test, I concluded that he had no weakness in either leg, and a sensitivity test showed intact sensation in both legs. There were no signs of a herniated disc or nerve impingement, no spinal fracture, no pain radiating to the legs, and no numbness or tingling sensations, so I concluded that Frank had an acute sprain in his lower back.

SYMPTOMS, CAUSES, AND DIAGNOSIS

Lumbar muscle strains and sprains are the most common causes of low back pain, and they occur when the muscles or fibers are abnormally stretched or torn. Ligaments torn from their attachments are the cause of a lumbar sprain, which does not show up on X-rays or an MRI. And because it can be difficult to differentiate between a sprain and a strain, the diagnosis of these two conditions is often confused.

The most important differentiations for acute lower back pain, as opposed to severe herniated discs or lower back nerve impingements, are that the latter two conditions involve the following.

- Loss of control of the bladder or bowels
- Numbness and tingling sensation in one or both legs
- Progressive weakness in the lower extremities
- Lower back pain radiating down one or both legs

If an acute low back pain is accompanied by these four symptoms, the patient likely has either a herniated disc or the lumbosacral nerves are impinged. If there is only acute lower back pain without these four symptoms, that indicates there is a sprain or strain in the lower back.

TREATMENTS FOR ACUTE LOW BACK SPRAIN IN WESTERN MEDICINE

Noninvasive Treatments

The treatments used for a lower back sprain and a herniated disc are different. For acute lower back sprain, the following methods are utilized.

Bed Rest

According to the protocols of Western medicine, bed rest is usually prescribed for a few days, up to one week. Doctors expect that their patients will feel better after bed rest and will be able to return to their work and daily functions. This treatment, however, is usually not very successful.

Medications

Western medicine also employs anti-inflammatory medications or muscle relaxants, though this treatment, too, is not usually successful in alleviating acute lower back pain.

A Lumbosacral Brace

Sometimes the patient is fitted with a brace—a lumbosacral corset that helps support the back—but there are side effects to using this because

a corset weakens the mus-
cles and ligaments of the
lower back.

Physical Therapy

Physical therapy can help
overcome the side effects of
the lumbosacral brace and
patients can learn to acti-

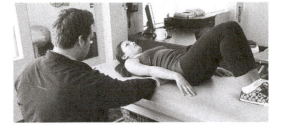

Figure 27.1

vate their own deep core muscles to protect their spine (see Figure 27.1).

TREATMENTS FOR ACUTE LOW BACK SPRAIN IN TRADITIONAL CHINESE MEDICINE

Acupuncture

Traditional Chinese medicine treats this condition with acupuncture. The acupuncture points used are Zan Zhu UB 2, Sheng Shu UB 23, Da Chang Shu UB 25, Huang Tiao GB 30, Wei Zhong UB 40, Cheng Shan UB 57, Kun Lun UB 60, and the Arshi points (the tender points along the lower back).

All these points except the GB 30 belong to the urinary bladder meridian. I usually start treatment by inserting the needles into the Zan Zhu UB 2 and asking the patient to stand up. Then I insert the needles deeply along the Zan Zhu and apply a strong stimulation, either manipulating the needles by hand or via an electrical stimulation. The energy of the stimulation should transmit from the needles and travel upward along the meridian of the bladder to the scalp, forehead, and back of the neck, and then down along the upper back and into the lower back and legs. I then ask the patient to gradually move his or her back forward and backward and then turn around. Many are afraid to do so because they think these movements will exacerbate the pain, but the energy stimulation should relax the lower back muscles and make movement easier.

Usually, acute stimulation of the needles for 15–20 minutes greatly improves the movement of the lower back and alleviates the pain, making the range of motion in this area much better. After the range of motion improves, the patient is asked to lie face down on the table. I then insert the needles into the local Arshi points (around the muscles that are spasming) and into UB 40, UB 57, and UB 60, and apply a strong electrical stimulation for 30 minutes. This should stimulate the entire bladder meridian and gradually relax the lower back muscles (see Table 27.1 and Figures 27.2 and 27.3).

Table 27.1

	Points	Meridian/Number	Location	Conditions Helped
1	Zan Zhu	UB 2	On the medial extremity of the eyebrow, or on the supraorbital notch	Headaches, blurring and failing of vision, pain above the eye, tearing, redness, swelling, and pain of the eye, twitching eyelids, glaucoma, acute lower back pain
2	Sheng Shu	UB 23	1.5 inches lateral to Mingmen (DU 4), at the level of the lower border of the spinous process of the 2nd lumbar vertebra	Nocturnal emissions, impotence, bedwetting, irregular menstruation, vaginal discharge, low back pain, weakness of the knee, blurred vision, dizziness, tinnitus, deafness, abdominal swelling, asthma, diarrhea
3	Da Chang Shu	UB 25	1.5 inches lateral to Yao Yang Guan (Du 3), at the level of the lower border of the spinous process of the 4th lumbar vertebra	Low back pain, intestinal gas, abdominal distension, diarrhea, constipation, muscular atrophy, pain, numbness, and motor impairment of the lower extremities, sciatica
4	Huan Tiao	GB 30	At the junction of the lateral 1/3 and medial 2/3 of the distance between the great trochanter and the hiatus of the sacrum (Yaoshu, Du 2); when locating the point, put the patient in lateral recumbent position with the thigh flexed.	Pain of the lumbar region and thigh, muscular atrophy of the lower limbs, paralysis on one side

(*Continued*)

Table 27.1 (*Continued*)

	Points	Meridian/ Number	Location	Conditions Helped
5	Wei Zhong	UB 40	Midpoint of the transverse crease of the popliteal fossa, between the tendons of the biceps femoris and semitendinosus muscles	Lower back pain, motor impairment of the hip joint, contracture of the tendons in the pit of the knee, muscular atrophy, pain, numbness, and motor impairment of the lower extremities, paralysis, abdominal pain, vomiting, diarrhea, skin infection
6	Cheng Shan	UB 57	Directly below the belly of the gastrocnemius muscle, on the line joining Wei Zhong UB 40 and the calcaneus tendon, about 8 inches below Wei Zhong UB 40	Lower back pain, spasm in the calf muscles, hemorrhoids, constipation, beriberi
7	Kun Lun	UB 60	In the depression between the external malleolus and calcaneus tendon	Headache, blurring of vision, neck rigidity, nosebleed, pain in the shoulder, back and arm, swelling and pain of the heel, difficult labor, epilepsy

FRANK'S TREATMENT

After the acupuncture treatment, Frank immediately felt a decrease in the intensity of the muscle spasms, and he was able to move his back and bend forward and backward to a regular position by 50 degrees. He went home, applied a heating pad to the affected area, and returned the following day for the same treatment, which decreased his pain by almost 100 percent. At this point, I prescribed a regimen of exercises and stretches that completely relieved the pain. This treatment is effective for both acute lower back strain and sprain.

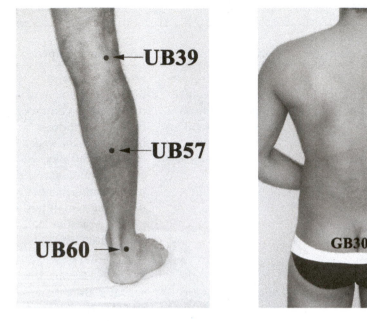

Figure 27.2   Figure 27.3

TIPS FOR PEOPLE WITH ACUTE LOW BACK SPRAIN

- If you feel the pain radiating to your legs, experience weakness, numbness, or a tingling sensation in your legs, you may have a herniated lumbosacral disc instead of acute lower back sprain.
- If you experience urinary incontinency, this is an indication that you have a herniated disc and it is affecting the nerves controlling your urinary system.
- If you have the previously mentioned symptoms, you must consult a physician and ask for an MRI to make a clear diagnosis.

TIPS FOR ACUPUNCTURE PRACTITIONERS

- You should always encourage your patients to move their backs during the stimulation of the Zan Zhu UB 2, even if they are afraid to do so.
- The stimulation should be strong—stronger than the pain the patient feels in the lower back.
- If you use a combined treatment of massage, acupuncture, and heating pads, you will have better results.
- Points in the UB meridian are the most important ones for treating acute low back pain.

28

Chronic Low Back Pain

Jason is a 46-year-old man who'd had low back pain on and off for about six months when he came to see me. He is a special education teacher who was able to catch a student who was falling and was about to hit the corner of a desk, but just as he did so, he felt the sudden onset of low back pain. The pain was so severe that Jason was unable to stand; he felt weak, and the pain was radiating to his left leg, causing a tingling and the sensation of numbness there. When he was brought to my office, he was unable to stand and had to talk to me from a prone position on the examining table.

About a year before that, Jason had had a similar experience with a student, and at that time, he had felt the same sensation of low back pain that radiated to his left leg, and was accompanied by tingling, tenderness, numbness, and heaviness of his left leg. After this incident, he had consulted his primary care physician, who diagnosed acute low back sprain, and prescribed anti-inflammatory medication and bed rest. After two days he felt a little better, but afterward he experienced off-and-on pain and a weak lower back.

When Jason came to see me, he found it difficult to bend his back forward and backward and hold up his low back. His left leg was heavy, and he had difficulty raising it. He could not bend forward with any ease and said he had trouble putting on his pants. He also had difficulty picking up objects from the floor, such as a pen, and was experiencing a bit of urinary incontinence.

Jason is moderately obese and has a somewhat large abdomen. When I asked him to stand straight and then bend forward, he was unable to perform the maneuver because he immediately felt a weakness in his back and had difficulty bending forward more than 40 degrees. I asked him to walk on his tiptoes and heels, but he was unable to do so. He reported that, when walking on his heels, he felt low back pain radiating down the left leg, especially around the knee and lower leg. I also tried to raise his legs straight—on the right side, he could do a straight-leg raise to about 80 degrees, but on the left side he could only do 50 degrees, at which point he felt the pain again radiating down to the leg and knee. I used a pinprick to check his response to sharpness and a cotton ball to check his ability to feel a light touch, and both tests showed decreased sensation along the left thigh and leg. I also found weakness in his left leg, knee, and ankle.

Because of the severity of Jason's condition, I ordered a lumbosacral MRI that showed a severe L4/L5 herniated disc protruding from the left side of the spine (see Figures 28.1 and 28.2).

From these MRI pictures, you can see that the arrows indicate the herniated disc in Jason's lumbar spine. Jason appeared to have left L5 radiculopathy, and because the images showed a severe herniated disc between L4 and L5, he was immediately referred to a neurosurgeon. After careful examination by a neurosurgeon, he was advised to have an emergency discectomy. This is a small incision to cut off part of his herniated disc; it is based on his emergency symptoms, such as severe low back pain radiating to his left leg with numbness and a tingling sensation, and a slight urinary incontinency.

Jason agreed to the surgery, but both his insurance companies argued against it, preventing him from going ahead with it immediately. While at work waiting for approval for the surgery, he went through two similar episodes of the same low back injury described earlier, and the second workers' compensation company requested that the first workers' compensation company pay the medical expenses because they believed the second injury was the consequence of Jason's first injury, but the first workers' compensation company refused the request. Nobody, it seems, wanted to pay the expenses, and Jason was in so much pain that he could not wait for the final decision between the two companies,

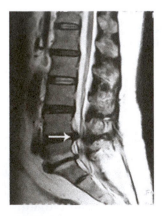

Figure 28.1

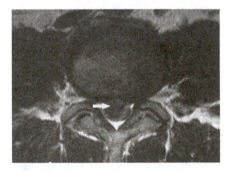

Figure 28.2

which he thought could take months. He called me and said, "I am stuck here, nobody wants to pay for the surgery, so I can't have it now. Could you please help me with acupuncture, so I can avoid the surgery if possible?" I decided to accept the challenge and started treating him right away.

SYMPTOMS, CAUSES, AND DIAGNOSIS

Low back pain is the second most common injury responsible for loss of working time in the United States, and almost everyone has experienced this kind of pain sometime in his or her life.

Low back pain has many different manifestations, the causes of which include the following.

- Myofascial or tendon ligament sprain. This acute pain in the muscles can come from poor posture, tendon ligament injury, overuse, or overstretching.
- Radiculopathy is a pinched nerve that usually originates from a herniated (slipped) disc pinching one of the lumbosacral roots, as indicated in Jason's MRI pictures.
- Spinal stenosis and narrowing of the nerve opening, either around the spinal cord or nerve roots, causes symptoms similar to a pinched nerve.
- Overuse and overstretching of ligaments of the facet and sacroiliac joints.
- Fracture of the vertebrae, caused by a significant force, such as an automobile or bicycle accident, or a fall.
- Scoliosis or kyphosis, where the spine curves.
- A compression fracture, which is common among postmenopausal women with osteoporosis.

There are also some less common spinal conditions capable of causing low back pain, including the following.

- Ankylosing spondylitis, which is a severe bony fusion of the lumbosacral spine and pelvic bone, with unknown causes. People with this condition have difficulty straightening their backs and are sometimes unable to look at the sky.
- Bacterial infections, such as osteomyelitis.
- Spinal tumors.
- Paget disease, which is a bone disease where the bone is unable to lay down new bone and take up old bone for the purpose of

rebuilding. As a result, the bone formation is abnormal, with loose bone structure and enlarged low-density bones that are brittle and prone to fracturing.

- Scheuermann's disease, a condition where the bones of the spinal vertebrae develop wedge-shaped deformities. As the vertebrae grow unevenly, the anterior angle is often greater than the posterior angle, and this results in the wedging shape of the vertebrae and curving of the spine.

The symptoms and a physical exam usually point toward the correct diagnosis. However, to be sure, it is important to also have the following tests performed.

- X-rays of the area will give evidence of lumbosacral osteoarthritis, sacroiliac osteoarthritis, and any degenerative changes of the disc.
- An MRI will indicate the herniated disc, nerve impingement, and facet joint osteoarthritis in the spine, and will also give a clear view of any degenerative changes of the disc.
- Electromyography, which is divided into two parts.

  - The first part is a nerve conduction study in which electrical stimulation is used to stimulate the nerves in one extremity. The machine then checks the velocity of the nerve's travel and the amplitude of each individual nerve, and that is compared to the opposite, or paired, extremity. If there is any difference in the velocity and amplitude, it is possible to differentiate among the nerves and determine which ones are injured.
  - The second part consists of an electromyography, during which a small needle is inserted into certain muscles of the spine and extremities. If the muscle is injured, it will show up on the screen, and this will pinpoint the nerve roots that are injured.

- Lumbar myography. This is radiographic examination of the lumbar spinal canal with an intrathecal injection of contrast medium. After the injection, X-rays are taken, which will show if any nerve roots are impinged.

Based on clinical symptoms and a physical examination, plus one or all of the tests discussed earlier, a clear diagnosis of lower back pain can be made.

TREATMENTS FOR CHRONIC LOW BACK PAIN IN WESTERN MEDICINE

Generally speaking, there are two major types of treatment for lower back pain, noninvasive and invasive.

Noninvasive Treatments

Most physicians recommend the following noninvasive treatments before resorting to surgery.

Medications

Anti-inflammatory drugs, such as acetaminophen, Advil, or naproxen, and muscle relaxants, such as Valium or Skelaxin, probably help relax lower back muscles.

Brace

For a more severe condition, a lumbosacral brace or binder is usually recommended to give support in the lower back. However, continued use of a brace can lead to muscle weakness in the lower back and should therefore be used only for such activities as driving, lifting a baby, or carrying a heavy object.

Traction

If the diagnosis is a herniated disc, the usual treatment would be traction. The patient is placed on a folding bed and then an attempt is made to pull the vertebrae slightly apart in order to allow the herniated disc to return to its original position. Traction is not indicated for other lower back pain, such as myofascial sprain, spinal stenosis, or spondylolisthesis, and the traction must be guided by a physician (see Figure 28.3).

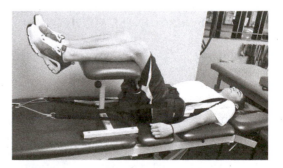

Figure 28.3

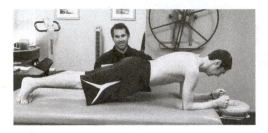

Figure 28.4

Physical Therapy

Physical therapy helps strengthen the abdominal and leg muscles, which will alleviate the back pain. A strong abdominal muscle helps hold the entire trunk (see Figure 28.4).

Invasive Treatments

Epidural Injections

If the noninvasive treatments do not help, then epidural injections are indicated. Epidural injections under fluoroscope, and X-ray-guided injections of steroids and lidocaine into the facet joint or nerve root, do decrease the inflammation in the nerve root, as well as the pain.

Surgery

Surgery is the last resort, and there are several surgical options.

> *discectomy* surgically cuts into the herniated disc to decrease the compression of the nerve root.
>
> *laminectomy* is used if the discectomy is not successful; in this surgery, a piece of the bone is removed to release the impinged nerve root.
>
> *Fusion.* If the vertebral body is unsteady and cannot hold together, it is necessary to use a rod or bone chip to fuse the vertebrae, which protects the nerve from further impingement.

TREATMENTS FOR CHRONIC LOW BACK PAIN IN TRADITIONAL CHINESE MEDICINE

Acupuncture

All the acupuncture points chosen are along the nerve distribution in the spine, and it is typical to stimulate these points with electrical stimulation combined with moxibustion and massage, all of which done together greatly help.

Hua Tuo Jia Ji points (see Figure 28.5) are sets of specially designed points used to treat disc disease. The acupuncturist should feel the herniated disc in the spine, the most tender points along the spine and then insert the needles around the herniated disc for a total of nine needles, as indicated in Figure 28.5.

Table 28.1

	Points	Meridian/ Number	Location	Conditions Helped
1	Hua Tuo Jia Ji	Experienced Points	Along the spine, use the most painful vertebral spinal as midpoint, then locate the upper and lower spinal process; 0.5 inches on either side you may choose two spinal process as the starting points. *See* Figure 28.5	Specific treatment for local neck and low back pain, and pain along the spine
2	Sheng Shu	UB 23	1.5 inches lateral to midline of spine at the level of the lower border of the spinous process of the 2nd lumbar vertebra	Nocturnal emissions, impotence, bedwetting, irregular menstruation, vaginal discharge, low back pain, weakness of the knee, blurring of vision, dizziness, tinnitus, deafness, swelling, asthma, diarrhea
3	Qi Hai Shu	UB 24	1.5 inches lateral to midline of spine at the level of the lower border of the spinous process of the 3rd lumbar vertebra	Low back pain, irregular or painful menstruation, asthma
4	Zhi Bian	UB 54	Lateral to the hiatus of the sacrum, 3 inches lateral to the midline of the spine	Pain in the lumbosacral region, muscular atrophy, motor impairment of the lower extremities, painful urination, swelling around external genitalia, hemorrhoids, constipation
5	Huan Tiao	GB 30	At the junction of the lateral 1/3 between the great trochanter and the hiatus of the sacrum	Pain in the lumbar region and thigh, muscular atrophy of the lower limbs, paralysis

(Continued)

Table 28.1   (*Continued*)

	Points	Meridian/ Number	Location	Conditions Helped
6	Yang Ling Quan	GB 34	In the depression anterior and inferior to the head of the fibula	Weakness, paralysis, numbness, and pain of the knee, beriberi, bitter taste in the mouth, vomiting, jaundice, infantile convulsions
7	Jue Gu (Xuan Zhong)	GB 39	3 inches above the tip of the external malleolus, in the depression between the posterior border of the fibula and the tendons of peroneus longus and brevis	Apoplexy, paralysis pain of the neck, abdominal distension, abdominal pain, muscular atrophy of the lower limbs, spastic pain of the leg, beriberi
8	Cheng Fu	UB 36	In the middle of the transverse gluteal fold	Pain in the lower back and gluteal region, constipation, muscular atrophy, pain, numbness, and motor impairment of the lower extremities

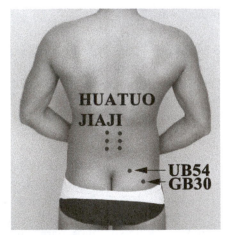

Figure 28.5

JASON'S TREATMENT

I treated Jason with a combination of both Western and Chinese medicines. I first inserted the needles into L4 and extended the Hua Tuo Jia Ji with nine needles to the L3 and L5 levels. I also selected UB 23 Sheng Shu, UB 24 Qi Hai Shu, UB 54 Zhi Bian, GB 30 Huan Tiao, GB 34 Yang Ling Quan, GB 39 Jue Gu, and UB 36 Cheng Fu.

In addition to acupuncture, I used a heating pad, massages, and 20 minutes of a traction machine for 90 pounds to stabilize his lower back. I prescribed a customized lumbosacral corset (a back brace), and treated him three times a week for eight weeks.

As the pain gradually subsided, Jason felt less weakness in his leg, and the burning and tingling sensations went away, so he was able to return to work. He continued seeing me for maintenance visits every two weeks and then once a month. After six months, he went back to the neurosurgeon. who decided that, based on the low intensity of his lower back pain, surgery was no longer indicated. Thanks to my treatments, Jason's back once again felt normal, and he continued to be pain free.

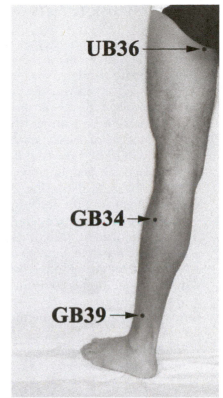

TIPS FOR PEOPLE WITH CHRONIC LOW BACK PAIN

Figure 28.6

- Identifying the symptoms is very important.
- If you feel your low back pain radiating down to the leg and there is numbness, a tingling sensation, and weakness, sometimes accompanied with slightly urinary incontinency, you need to have your doctor order an MRI to make a clear diagnosis.
- If the problem is acute or chronic low back sprain, you may need a few acupuncture treatments with massages and a heating pad. If it is pinched nerves in the lower back with the above symptoms, you should ask your acupuncturist to use Hua Tuo Jia Ji points, accompanied with massages, a heating pad, and even a traction machine for 20 minutes.
- A brace for the lower back always helps reduce your pain. However, because of the side effects, you cannot use it 24 hours a day. If you use it for too long a time, it can weaken your lower back and your abdominal muscles. You can use it only intermittently, no longer than two hours at a time.

TIPS FOR ACUPUNCTURISTS

- It is absolutely necessary to make a clear diagnosis. Differentiate acute and chronic lower back pain and differentiate muscle sprain from a herniated disc, a spinal stenosis and a radiculopathy because only in this way can the prognosis be accurately predicted. For example, if the diagnosis is a muscle spasm, acupuncture can greatly lessen the pain and help the patient experience a quick recovery so he or she can most probably return to work after only one or two days. However, if the patient has a herniated disc or spinal stenosis, acupuncture will probably help, but it will be a long recovery, in all likelihood two or three months.
- Most patients opt for nonsurgical treatment first. However, if the pain radiates down the leg, with numbness and tingling combined with urinary incontinence, it is very important to have an MRI and CT scan or X-ray to first make sure there is no significant herniated disc, or spondylolisthesis, or spinal stenosis. If a severe medical condition is confirmed, then it is best to refer the patient to a neurosurgeon.
- Acupuncture can treat a herniated disc, especially if it is combined with traction and massages.
- A lumbosacral corset is also a great tool for helping a patient move around with less pain.

29

Low Back Pain with Failed Back Surgery Syndrome (FBSS)

Peter is a 56-year-old man who complained of low back pain for three years. His pain started in the low back and radiated down to the right leg, which made sitting, walking, and standing difficult. The pain also interfered with his sleep, especially when he changed positions in the bed, prompting him to visit his primary care physician, who referred him to physical therapy. He did therapy for about three months, but the pain was not getting any better and he still felt constant sharp and stabbing pain that radiated down to the right lateral thigh and lower leg. During this time, he gradually felt his leg weakening and he had difficulty standing up from the sitting and driving position.

Then one day, Peter realized his underwear was wet because he had difficulty controlling his bladder. He also had a decreased sensation in his right lateral lower leg, so his primary care physician referred him to a neurosurgeon. An MRI was done, which showed two large right L4/L5 and L5/S1 herniated discs, and he was advised to have an L5/S1 discectomy.

He was afraid of the surgery, so he consulted another neurosurgeon, who suggested a laminectomy because the MRI showed two levels, L5 and S1, with nerve impingement and degenerative changes between L5 and S1 and S1 and S2, the reasons for his urinary incontinence.

He decided to wait a few more months to see if this would get better. He restarted physical therapy and had an epidural injection, and his pain seemed slightly better. But he still felt the right leg was weaker, and he sometimes lost control of his urine, so he decided to have surgery.

A laminectomy was performed, and one month after the surgery, Peter felt relief from his pain and could control his urine and bowel movements. He was very happy about the surgery.

Six months later, however, he started to feel low back pain again, and this time he felt the pain as a gradual onset, dull and achy, with no radiating down to the leg and no bowel or bladder abnormalities. There was, however, some weakness, and a mild numbness and tingling sensation on the right leg, so he visited his neurosurgeon, who told him this pain sometimes occurs about six months after surgery, and if he continued to do the physical therapy, it should get better.

Peter started the physical therapy again, doing muscle strengthening and stretching his lower back. However, one day, the pain suddenly got worse after waking up. It was like a stabbing and burning sensation around the L3/L4, L5/S1 middle spine, and from then on he experienced difficulty bending forward and backward, sitting to standing, and driving. He revisited his surgeon and was prescribed Tylenol with Codeine. This pain medication made him feel better, but he started getting drowsy and had difficulty driving and concentrating on his work. He also gradually started craving this drug. If he did not take it for one day, he felt uncomfortable, not only in the lower back but also in the entire body, and he was also depressed and had low energy. At this point, he was desperate and came to me for evaluation and treatment.

I performed a physical examination and saw the scars on both sides of the spine. When I touched him, there was tenderness in the spine but no tenderness in the sciatic region. He could bend his low back forward only about 40 degrees and backward only about 10 degrees, but he had no problem walking on tippy toes and heels, and had no decreased sensation in his legs. I compared his pre-surgery and post-surgery MRIs and found no impingement of the nerve roots. Based on all this information, I decided that Peter had a condition called post-lumbosacral laminectomy syndrome, also known as failed back surgery syndrome (FBSS), which refers to chronic back and/or leg pain that occurs after spinal surgery.

SYMPTOMS, CAUSES, AND DIAGNOSIS

Surgeries That Could Result in FBSS

Before discussing FBSS, I would like to elaborate on the basics of the seven types of low back surgery that could result in FBSS: discectomy, foraminotomy, intradiscal electrothermal therapy, nucleoplasty, radiofrequency, spinal fusion, and spinal laminectomy.

> *A discectomy* is a procedure done to relieve pressure on a nerve root that's being compressed by a bulging disc or bone spur. In order to relieve this pressure, the surgeon removes a small piece of the lamina (the bony roof of the spinal canal) from above the obstruction. (See Figure 29.1.)

A foraminotomy is surgery undertaken to enlarge the foramen (the bony hole), where a nerve root branches out from the spinal canal. Joints thickened with age, or bulging discs, may cause the foramen to narrow and thereby press on the nerve. This pressure can cause pain, numbness, or weakness in the extremities. In order to relieve the pressure, the surgeon removes small pieces of bone over the nerve through a small slit, which allows her or him to cut away the blockage. (See Figure 29.2.)

Nucleoplasty is used to treat lower back pain resulting from mildly herniated discs. During this procedure, a wandlike instrument is guided by X-ray imaging and inserted through a needle into the disc in order to create a channel. This facilitates the removal of inner disc material. Several channels may be made, depending on the amount of material that needs to be removed. After removal, the wand heats and shrinks the tissue of the disc wall in order to seal it. (See Figure 29.3.)

Radiofrequency (RF) lessening is a procedure used to interrupt nerve conduction and the transfer of pain signals. Electrical impulses are used in order to destroy the nerves located in the affected area. A special needle is inserted into the localized nerve tissue, with the guidance of an X-ray. This area is then heated for 90–120 seconds, destroying the nerve tissue. This can help stop pain for 6–12 months. (See Figure 29.4.)

Spinal fusion is a procedure that is done in order to support a weak spine and/or to prevent painful movements. However, spinal fusion requires a long recovery period and may result in a permanent loss of spinal flexibility. The procedure involves the removal of the spinal disc between two vertebrae, and the subsequent fusion of those vertebrae. Methods of fusion include either bone grafting and/or using metal devices secured by screws. (See Figure 29.5.)

Spinal laminectomy is a procedure done to relieve pressure on the spinal cord and nerve roots. Also known as spinal decompression, this type of surgery involves the removal of the lamina to increase the size of the spinal canal.

Symptoms and Causes of FBSS

FBSS is characterized by intractable, diffuse, dull, and aching pain, or sharp, pricking, and stabbing pain in the back and/or legs, accompanied by varying degrees of functional incapacitation. A recurrent herniated disc and symptomatic hypertrophic scar—the result of over-healing, where the body produces too much connective tissue too quickly, causing a larger, more noticeable scar—can produce low back symptoms and radiculopathy similar to those before the surgery. Gradually increasing symptoms beginning a year or more after a discectomy are considered more likely a result of scar radiculopathy, while a more abrupt onset at any interval after surgery is more likely due to a recurrent herniated disc. Multiple factors can contribute to the onset or development of FBSS, such as residual or recurrent disc herniation, persistent postoperative pressure on a spinal nerve, altered joint mobility, double-jointedness with instability, scar tissue (fibrosis), depression, anxiety, sleeplessness, and spinal muscular deconditioning.

In 1992, the journal *Spine* published a survey of 74 journal articles that reported the results after decompression for spinal stenosis. On average, good to excellent results were reported by 64 percent of the patients, which left about 36 percent of the post-back-surgery patients who experienced some degree of back pain, usually six months after surgery. For some, the pain could achieve pre-operation intensity two years after the surgery.[1]

TREATMENTS FOR FBSS IN WESTERN MEDICINE

Noninvasive Treatments

The treatments for FBSS in Western medicine include physical therapy, minor nerve blocks, transcutaneous electrical nerve stimulation (TENS), behavioral medicine, nonsteroidal anti-inflammatory (NSAID) medications, membrane stabilizers, antidepressants, and intrathecal morphine pump. Six of these treatments are discussed next.

Physical Therapy

Spinal surgery changes the anatomy of the spine but does nothing to improve the activation of deep-core stabilizing muscles. One of the benefits of physical therapy for retraining the body is to properly activate the deep-core muscles that stabilize the spine. The two deep co-stabilizing muscles of the spine are the transverse abdominis (TrA) and the multifidus.

Spinal Braces

These are an option, especially when worn to improve recovery immediately following the surgery. A corset helps to brace the lumbar spine by increasing the pressure in the abdomen, thereby reducing the amount of weight placed on the spine. The transverse abdominis, often called the human corset, is the only abdominal muscle that attaches to the posterior spine and runs transverse around the body.

Quadruped Exercises

Quadruped alternating UE/LE movement is also called bird-dog, while dead-bug is the name of supine alternating UE/LE movement. It is important to maintain a neutral spine from hips to shoulders, and for the core to take in the force when an extremity is lifted, and not involve a rotation component to the opposite hand or knee. This will occur if done improperly or rushed to without developing strength and control through the previously mentioned exercises.

Both the bird-dog and dead-bug can be progressed from a solid stable surface, such as the ground or an exercise mat, to an unstable surface, such as foam DynaDisc or a foam roller, to increase the activation of core-stabilizing muscles, thereby making the exercise more challenging and effective. (See Figures 29.1 and 29.2.)

Soft-Tissue Mobilization

Adhesions and scar-tissue are very common following

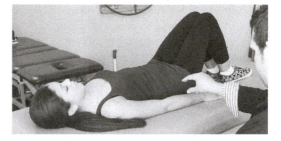

Figure 29.1

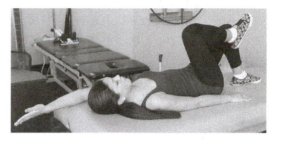

Figure 29.2

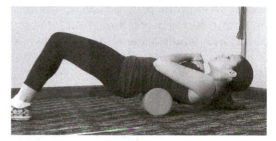

Figure 29.3

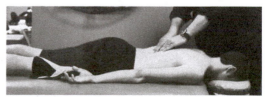

Figure 29.4

any surgery. Development of these adhesions can lead to decreased mobility and compression on nerve roots, causing increased stiffness and pain. A few simple techniques to rid adhesions/trigger points/scar tissue and improve recovery along the spine can come from using a foam roller or having manual work specific to your individual needs. (See Figures 29.3 and 29.4.)

Medications

Acetaminophen

Tylenol (one brand name) helps many kinds of chronic pain. NSAIDs also help with pain conditions. Examples include aspirin, ibuprofen (two brand names: Motrin, Advil), and naproxen (one brand name: Aleve). NSAIDs come in both over-the-counter and prescription forms. These medicines can be taken just when you need them, or they can be taken every day. When these medicines are taken regularly, they build up to levels in the blood that fight the pain of inflammation (swelling), and also give general pain relief. It is important to always take NSAIDs with food or milk because the most common negative side effects are related to the stomach.

Narcotics can be addictive. For many with severe chronic pain, these drugs are an important part of their therapy. If your doctor prescribes narcotics for your pain, be sure to carefully follow his or her directions. Tell your doctor if you are uncomfortable with the changes that may go along with taking these medicines, such as the inability to concentrate or think clearly. Do not drive or operate heavy machinery when taking these drugs. When you're taking narcotics, it's important to know that there is a difference between physical dependence and psychological addiction. Physical dependence on a medicine means your body gets used to that medicine and needs it in order to work properly. Psychological addiction is the desire to use a drug whether or not it's needed to relieve pain. Narcotic drugs often cause constipation (difficulty having bowel movements). If you are taking a narcotic medicine, it's important to drink at least six to eight glasses of water every day, and try to eat two to four servings of fresh fruits and three to five servings of vegetables every day.

Other Medicines

Many drugs that are used to treat other illnesses can also treat pain. For example, carbamazepine (Neurontin) is a seizure medicine that can also treat some kinds of pain. Amitriptyline is an antidepressant that can also help with chronic pain. It can take several weeks before these medicines begin to work well.

Transcutaneous Electrical Nerve Stimulation (TENS)

TENS is thought to disrupt the pain being transmitted to the brain by delivering a different, non-painful, sensation to the skin around the pain site. In essence, it modulates the way the body processes the pain sensations from that area—it closes the pain gate to the brain. It can also trigger the brain to release endorphins that act as natural painkillers, and help promote a feeling of well-being. (See Figure 29.5.)

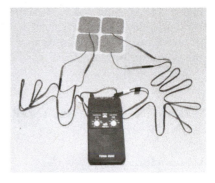

Figure 29.5

Invasive Treatments

Local Nerve Block

Epidural steroid injections may be minimally helpful in some cases. An epidural nerve block is the injection of corticosteroid medication into the epidural space of the spinal column. This space is located between the dura (a membrane surrounding the nerve roots) and the interior surface of the spinal canal formed by the vertebrae.

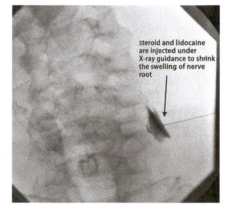

steroid and lidocaine are injected under X-ray guidance to shrink the swelling of nerve root

Figure 29.6

After a local skin anesthetic is applied to numb the injection site, a spinal needle is inserted into the epidural space under fluoroscopic (X-ray) guidance, using a contrast agent to confirm needle placement. Local anesthetic and corticosteroid anti-inflammatory medication are delivered into the epidural space to shrink the swelling around nerve roots, relieving pressure and pain. (See Figure 29.6.)

Intrathecal Morphine Pump

Pain-pump delivery of narcotic drugs is a rather new option available to those with cancer (and non-cancer) pain. It is also called intraspinal (within the spine) or intrathecal (within the spinal canal) delivery. It was first used in 1979 after the discovery of narcotic receptors in the spinal cord. The use of an implant device to deliver medications directly in the area of the spinal cord was first used in 1981 for cancer pain. Since then, the pain pump has been used for chronic non-cancer pain, such as failed low back surgery syndrome and such neurological conditions as cerebral palsy, multiple sclerosis, or spinal cord injury.

TREATMENTS FOR FBSS IN TRADITIONAL CHINESE MEDICINE

Acupuncture

According to traditional Chinese medicine, there are three types of FBSS.

Type 1. Coldness and Wetness of FBSS

Patients feel cold and heavy; there is pain in the entire low back, difficulty turning over in bed, or standing up from a sitting position, and this becomes worse in cold weather, when stiffness in the low back, hip, and knee joints develops.

Acupuncture points are UB 25 Da Chang Shu, GB 30 Huan Tiao, UB 40 Wei Zhong, UB 60 Kun Lun, plus Du 26 Ren Zhong, GB 34 Yang Ling Quan, and UB 58 Fei Yang (see Figures 29.7 to 29.11 and Table 29.1).

Type 2. Kidney Deficiency of FBSS

Weakness and pain in nonspecific areas, difficulty standing, feeling better when lying in bed, dull, achy pain and cold in the four extremities.

Acupuncture points are UB 25 Da Chang Shu, GB 30 Huan Tiao, UB 40 Wei Zhong, UB 60 Kun Lun, plus St 36 Zu San Li, Sp 6 San Yin Jiao, and Ki 3 Tai Xi (see Table 29.2).

Type 3. Blood Stagnation of FBSS

There is sharp, stabbing pain in specific areas of the low back and buttocks—the pain is so severe that nobody can touch the tender area. There is difficulty bending, sitting, standing, and turning over in bed.

Acupuncture points: UB 25 Da Chang Shu, GB 30 Huan Tiao, UB 40 Wei Zhong, UB 60 Kun Lun, plus Sp 10 Xue Hai, UB 17 Ge Shu, LI 4 He Gu, and UB 57 Cheng Shan (see Table 29.3).

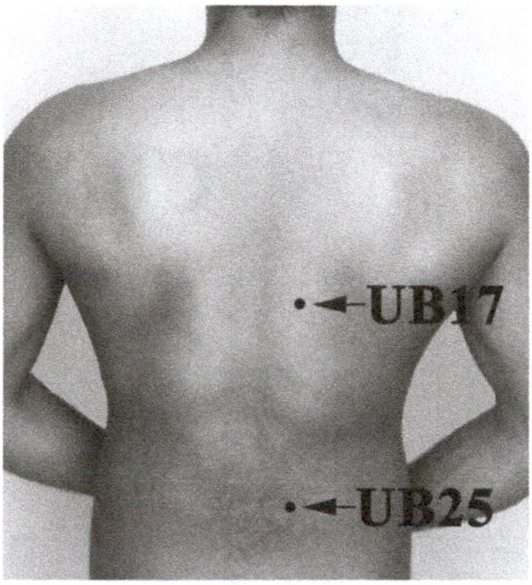

Figure 29.7

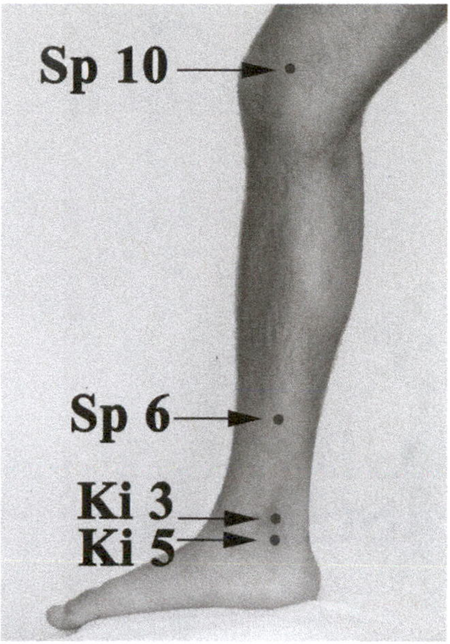

Figure 29.8

PETER'S TREATMENT

Peter underwent treatment with both acupuncture and physical therapy. The typical protocol included heat, massage, and acupuncture, in that order. Peter was first put on the bed with a heating pad on his lower back for about 10–15 minutes, to gradually loosen the muscles of his lower back; then a massage was given to further relax these muscles.

After the massage came the acupuncture treatment, and the most important points were selected based on the above principle. He was given needles with electrical stimulation for 20–30 minutes, to activate his flow of energy and gradually decrease the pain.

He then was transferred to the physical therapy area, where he was guided to strengthen his abdominal and low back muscles.

He was given the above treatment for about 20 sessions, after which he felt great improvement—much more flexibility and much less pain. He has now been pain-free for a long time, and sometimes returns to my office for tune-ups.

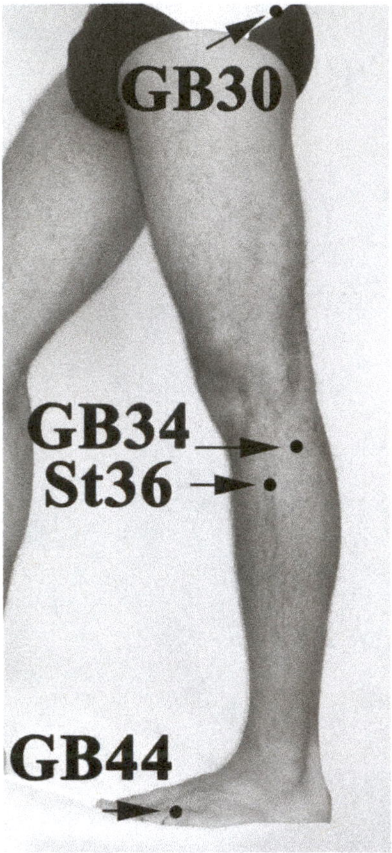

GB30

GB34
St36

GB44

Figure 29.9

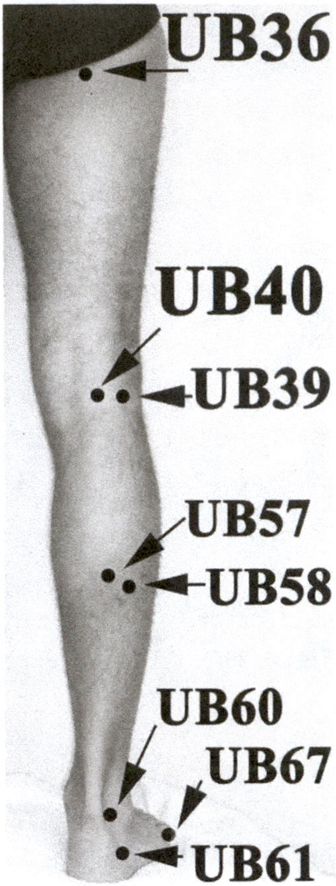

UB36

UB40
UB39

UB57
UB58

UB60
UB67
UB61

Figure 29.10

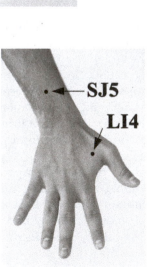

SJ5
LI4

Figure 29.11

Table 29.1.

	Points	Meridian/ Number	Location	Conditions Helped
1	Da Chang Shu	UB 25	1.5 inches lateral to midline of the body on the back, at the level of the spinous process of the 4th lumbar vertebra; see Figure 29.7.	Low back pain, abdominal distension, diarrhea, constipation, muscular atrophy, pain, numbness, and weakness in the legs, sciatica
2	Huan Tiao	GB30	At the junction of the lateral 1/3 and medial 2/3 of the distance between the great trochanter and the hiatus of the sacrum; see Figure 29.9.	Low back pain, thigh pain, muscular atrophy of the lower limbs, paralysis
3	Wei Zhong	UB 40	Midpoint of the transverse crease of the popliteal fossa, between the tendons of biceps femoris and semitendinosus muscles; see Figure 29.10.	Low back pain, motor impairment of the hip joint, muscular atrophy, pain, numbness, and motor impairment of the lower extremities, paralysis, abdominal pain, vomiting, diarrhea
4	Kun Lun	UB 60	In the depression between the external malleolus and calcaneus tendon; see Figure 29.10.	Headaches, blurring of vision, neck rigidity, nosebleed, pain in the shoulder, back, and arm, swelling and pain of the heel, difficult labor, epilepsy
5	Ren Zhong	Du 26	A little above the midpoint of the philtrum, near the nostrils; see Figure 29.11.	Mental disorders, epilepsy, hysteria, infantile convulsion, coma, deviation of the mouth and eyes, puffiness of the face, low back pain and stiffness

(Continued)

Table 29.1 *(Continued)*

	Points	Meridian/ Number	Location	Conditions Helped
6	Fei Yang	UB 58	7 inches directly above Kun Lun on the posterior border of fibula, about 1 inch inferior and lateral to Cheng Shan (UB 57); *see* Figure 29.10.	Headaches, blurring of vision, nasal obstruction, nosebleed, back pain, hemorrhoids, leg weakness

Table 29.2

	Points	Meridian/ Number	Location	Conditions Helped
1	Zu San Li	St 36	One finger-breadth from the anterior crest of the tibia in tibialis anterior muscle *See* Figure 29.9.	Gastric pain, vomiting, hiccups, abdominal distension, diarrhea, dysentery, constipation, knee joint and leg pain, edema, cough, asthma, poor digestion, dizziness, insomnia, mania
2	San Yin Jiao	Sp 6	3 inches directly above the tip of the medial malleolus, on the posterior border of the medial aspect of the tibia *See* Figure 29.8.	Abdominal pain, distension, diarrhea, irregular menstruation, uterine bleeding, prolapse of the uterus, sterility, delayed labor, night bedwetting, impotence, edema, hernia, pain in the external genitalia, muscular atrophy, motor impairment, paralysis and leg pain, headaches, dizziness, and vertigo, insomnia

(Continued)

184

Table 29.2 *(Continued)*

	Points	Meridian/ Number	Location	Conditions Helped
3	Tai Xi	Ki 3	In the depression between the medial malleolus and tendo calcaneus, at the level of the tip of the medial malleolus; *see* Figure 29.8.	Sore throat, toothache, deafness, tinnitus, dizziness, spitting up blood, asthma, thirst, irregular menstruation, insomnia, impotence, low back pain

Table 29.3

	Points	Meridian/ Number	Location	Conditions Helped
1	Xue Hai	Sp 10	2 inches above the medial superior border of the patella (knee-cap); *see* Figure 29.8.	Irregular menstruation, uterine bleeding, eczema, pain in the thigh
2	Ge Shu	UB 17	1.5 inches lateral to the middle line of the body on the back, at the level of the lower border of the spinous process of the 7th thoracic vertebra; *see* Figure 29.7.	Vomiting, hiccups, belching, difficulty in swallowing, asthma, cough, spitting up blood, afternoon fever, night sweating, measles
3	He Gu	LI 4	On the dorsum of the hand between the 1st and 2nd metacarpal bones, approximately in the middle of the 2nd metacarpal bone on the radial side; *see* Figure 29.12.	Headaches, pain in the neck, redness, swelling, and pain in the eye, nosebleed nasal obstruction, toothache, deafness, swelling of the face, sore throat, facial paralysis, abdominal pain, dysentery, constipation, delayed labor, infantile convulsions, pain, weakness, and motor impairment in the upper limbs

(Continued)

Table 29.3 *(Continued)*

Points	Meridian/ Number	Location	Conditions Helped
4 Cheng Shan	UB 57	Directly below the belly of gastrocnemius muscle, on the line joining Wei Zhong UB40 and calcaneus tendon, about 8 inches below Wei Zhong UB40; *see* Figure 29.10.	Low back pain, hemorrhoids, constipation, beriberi

TIPS FOR PEOPLE WHO STILL FEEL LOW BACK PAIN AFTER SURGERY

- An MRI of the spine in the low back area is necessary to check any new injuries, such as a new herniated disc, any degenerative changes of other levels, any loosening of the screws, or spinal stenosis.
- Sometimes, you may be advised to have the second surgery for your low back, but be very cautious about undergoing any subsequent low back surgery. From my personal experience, I have not seen many successful cases after a second or even a third operation.
- Seek out a physiatrist MD who also practices acupuncture. Physiatrist MDs in the United States are trained in musculoskeletal medicine. They not only understand your problem but can also, more specifically, treat you with acupuncture. They can also guide your physical therapist in your treatment.
- The combination of physical therapy, massages, and acupuncture is very important because these combined treatments not only relax your muscles but also maximize your ability to perform core body strengthening.
- Different people like different sequences of treatment. It is not absolutely necessary for you to have heat, massage, acupuncture, then physical therapy, because everybody is different. It depends on your personal preference. The most important thing is to have the combined treatment that benefits you the most.
- If you drive longer than 30 minutes, it is wise to wear the low back brace as it will protect your low back and prevent further injuries.

TIPS FOR ACUPUNCTURE PRACTITIONERS

- You must clearly understand the patient's pathological mechanism. Some patients are not allowed to have flexion exercise, and some patients cannot have extension exercise.
- A heating pad and a massage are both very important to induce energy and relax the low back muscles.
- LI 4 is a very important point, as per the gate theory, to increase the secretion of endorphins and inhibit the upgoing reticular formation that sends the pain signal to the brain, therefore altering the pain sensation sent to the brain.
- Electrical stimulation on the back points is a must.

30

Low Back Pain—Spinal Compression Fracture

Betty is a 70-year-old woman who complained of low back pain the day after she bent down to pick up her one-year-old granddaughter. Although she had no history of low back pain before this, she felt a spasm of sudden-onset low back pain and was unable to bend forward or move her back. She had difficulty sitting and standing, and the only position she felt comfortable in was lying down on the bed. She called her daughter right away and was put on bed rest. Betty thought she might have a low back sprain and would get better after being in bed overnight, but when she still felt the sharp, stabbing pain on the second day and could not move, she was brought to me for evaluation and treatment.

When I inquired into her pain, she reported that it was constant, especially in the right hip, and was accompanied by a stomach ache and slight shortness of breath, but she said there was no pain radiating down to her legs, no urinary or bowel incontinency, and no numbness or tingling sensation. Betty did have a 20-year history of osteoporosis and had been advised to take vitamin D (400 units) and calcium (800 mg) daily, but she frequently forgot to take them. She does exercise, swimming daily and using a stationary bike once or twice a week.

My examination of her showed that she had kyphosis—her back curved on the right side of the spine and her muscles on that side of the back were very spasmodic. The muscles on the left side of the back were looser, making her look like a hunchback. As she had only indicated a vague area of the entire low back, I was not able to identify any specific spot on her back that felt pain; she did not have any abnormal sensations in either leg, but because of her pain, I could not check for muscle strength there or in her back.

Since these signs and symptoms indicated to me that she might have a spinal compression fracture, I immediately ordered a CT scan of her spine. It depicted the wedge-shaped vertebra shown in Figure 30.1 and confirmed my diagnosis of a spinal compression fracture in her lower back.

THE SYMPTOMS, CAUSES, AND DIAGNOSIS

The Major Symptoms of Spinal Compression Fracture

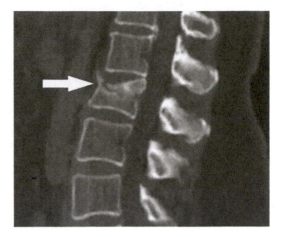

Figure 30.1

Most patients have sudden, severe back pain, worsening of pain when standing or walking, loss of height, deformity of the spine—a curved, hunchback shape, a feeling of relief from pain when lying down, and difficulty and pain when bending or twisting.

The neurological problems for this condition can manifest in many ways. An obvious problem is reduced leg strength or complete weakness. A loss of sensation in the lower extremities and the perianal area can be just as important, and urinary retention and urinary and fecal incontinence are very important signs that indicate the need for emergency surgery.

Most people with this set of symptoms were only doing slight activities before the pain started, such as getting in or out of a car, lifting a suitcase out of the trunk of a car, lifting a bag of groceries, getting up from a sitting position, bending to the floor to pick something up, lifting the corner of a mattress when changing bed linens, or they were involved in minor accidents, such as slipping on a rug or making a misstep.

The Primary Cause of Spinal Compression Fracture

The underlying cause of spinal compression fracture is osteoporosis. The vertebral bones lose their bone substance, and although the shape of the bones remains the same, they cannot hold the weight added to their body. The spongelike bone at the spine's low back cannot sustain any acute stress, such as a sudden bending forward to tie a shoelace or pick up something from the floor.

The reasons for osteoporosis are listed here.

- For women, the leading risk factors are menopause or estrogen deficiency, cigarette smoking, physical inactivity, use of prednisone, or poor nutrition.

- For men, low testosterone levels may be associated with osteoporosis, in addition to all the non-hormonal factors listed earlier.
- Renal or liver failure, which would cause nutritional deficiencies, and lead to decreased bone remodeling and increased osteopenia (borderline osteoporosis).
- Genetics. Osteoporosis can be observed in closely related family members.
- Malignant tumors, such as myelomas, lymphoma, or breast, lung, prostate, or renal cell cancers, could metastasize to the spine.
- Infections. Chronic osteomyelitis (bone infection) can result in spinal compression fracture.

Clues to Making a Diagnosis of Spinal Compression Fracture

Some people might have one or multiple spinal compression fractures without noticing them. However, by careful examination, a diagnosis can be made based on the following:

- The body might twist the spine to the side, leading to scoliosis.
- These fractures often create wedge-shaped vertebral bones, which make the spine bend forward. The curved back, or hunchback, is called kyphosis.
- Neck and back pain can eventually develop as your body tries to adapt to the postural changes in the spine.
- *Loss of height.* With each fracture of a spinal bone, the spine loses some of its height, and eventually, after several collapsed vertebrae, the person's shorter stature will be noticeable.
- *Hip pain.* The shorter spine brings the rib cage closer to the hip bones. If the rib and hip bones are rubbing against each other, there will be discomfort and pain.
- *Breathing problems.* If the spine becomes severely compressed, the lungs may not function properly and breathing problems, such as shortness of breath, can develop.
- Sometimes the poor spine position can make people prone to infections, such as bronchitis or pneumonia.
- *Stomach complaints.* A shorter spine can compress the stomach, and that can cause a bulging stomach and such digestive problems as acid reflux, constipation, poor appetite, or weight loss.

TREATMENTS FOR SPINAL COMPRESSION FRACTURE IN WESTERN MEDICINE

Noninvasive Treatments

The best treatment is prevention. All preventive measures should be taken, including such procedures as checking and correcting vision and hearing, evaluating any neurological problems, reviewing any prescription medications for side effects that may affect balance, and providing a checklist for improving safety at home.

Wearing undergarments with hip-pad protectors may prevent an injury to the hip in the event of a fall. Hip protectors may be considered for those with significant risk factors for falling, or those who have previously fractured a hip.

The use of tobacco or an excessive intake of alcohol is harmful. Alcohol and cigarettes inhibit osteoblast cell activities, which build up bone density, and improve the functioning of osteoclast cells, which usually destroy bone density.

Other methods of prevention include the use of supplements, medication, exercise, physical therapy, and braces.

Preventive Supplements

- Calcium, 1,000 mg a day for women before menopause, and 1,200 mg a day for women who are postmenopausal.
- Vitamin D, 800 IU a day for women before menopause, and 1,000 IU a day for postmenopausal women.
- Men up to the age of 50 should increase their vitamin D and calcium intake to 800 IU of vitamin D and 1,000 mg of calcium per day.

Preventive Medications

Bisphosphonates, such as alendronate (Fosamax), ibandronate (Boniva), risedronate (Actonel), and zoledronic acid (Reclast), slow the rate of bone thinning and can lead to increased bone density. These medicines can be used by men and women. (See also "Medications" section.)

Exercises

- Regular weight-bearing exercise. Weight-bearing exercise programs not only increase bone density but also improve both heart and lung functions and muscle strength. Walking with a one- to three-pound pound bag of sand tied on each calf for two to three miles a day will greatly improve your bone density if you stick to the program long enough.

- Increased walking, jogging, tai chi, stair climbing, dancing, and tennis.
- Muscle-strengthening exercises include weight training and other resistive exercises.

Physical Therapy

Recent research from astronauts, athletes, and those recovering from injury has shown many benefits of using a whole-body vibration (WBV) machine (see Figure 30.3) to increase strength and decrease bone-mineral-density losses. Holding a quarter-squat position for 30 seconds on a WBV, which helps the entire body exercise without an undue impact on the joints. A WBV is very effective for increasing BMD in postmenopausal women even in comparison to a walking regimen.[1]

Maintaining a neutral spine is very important, and you need to learn how to properly perform activities, such as getting in and out of bed while keeping your spine straight. This is accomplished by using a technique called the *log roll* to go from lying on your back with your knees bent to rolling onto your side, then pushing with your upper arm to a seated position, and finally to standing.

In addition to learning how to properly perform activities of daily living, such as getting in and out of bed, it is very important to work on core stabilizing, using the exercises described in Chapter 29 about low back pain with failed back surgery syndrome (see Figure 30.2).

Maintaining Balance

Performing a balance test, such as the Berg Balance test or the Tinetti test, will give you an objective measurement of your current balance level and risk of falls. Preventing the risk of falls is very crucial as low bone-density levels make fractures more likely.

There are many ways to improve balance, and there are progressions to help

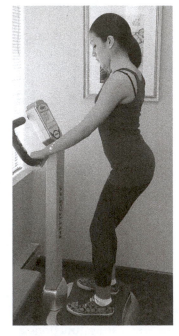

Figure 30.2

accomplish this. A basic progression is to place your feet at shoulder width and remain standing as long as you can. Stand in front of a counter or couch so you can use your hands to catch yourself if you experience a loss of balance, or better yet, have a spotter. Next assume a stance where one foot is in front of the other, as in a walking stride, and again work to balance yourself with your eyes open. Then narrow your stance until one foot is directly

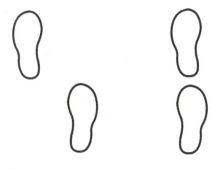

Figure 30.3

in front of the other in a heel-to-toe fashion called tandem stance. Once you are able to accomplish the tandem stance with your eyes open, go back to the walking-stride stance and work to the tandem stance with your eyes closed (see Figure 30.3).

Brace

Wearing a back brace is a very effective means of preventing unwarranted motions of the spine with a compression fracture pre- or post-surgery during early healing. Be cautious about wearing a brace for an extended period of time, typically more than six to eight weeks, to avoid any secondary complications of immobilization (see Figure 30.4).

Medications

Treatment of compression fractures is usually aimed at alleviating the pain and preventing injuries in the future.

A carefully prescribed cocktail of pain medications can relieve bone-on-bone, muscle, and nerve pain, explains F. Todd Wetzel, MD, professor of orthopedics and neurosurgery at Temple University School of Medicine in Philadelphia. "If it's prescribed correctly, you can reduce doses of the individual drugs in the cocktail."

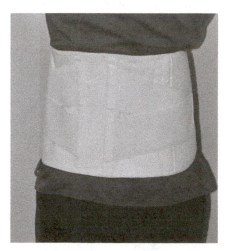

Figure 30.4

Over-the-counter pain medications are often sufficient to relieve pain. Two types of non-prescription medications—acetaminophen and nonsteroidal anti-inflammatory drugs—are recommended. Narcotic pain medications and muscle relaxants are often prescribed only for short periods of time, since there is a risk of addiction. Antidepressants can also help relieve nerve-related pain.

Invasive Treatment

Surgery

When chronic pain from a spinal compression fracture persists despite rest, activity modification, back bracing, and pain medication, surgery is the next step.

Surgical procedures used to treat spinal fractures include vertebroplasty, kyphoplasty, and spinal fusion surgery. If the pain is severe, and vertebral collapse is becoming problematic, vertebroplasty or kyphoplasty can be considered. In these surgical procedures, an interventional radiologist restores the height of the bone and injects cement into the vertebra to stabilize the fracture and prevent further collapse.

Vertebroplasty. After general anesthesia, or simply under sedation, a special bone needle guided by X-ray is inserted into the soft tissues of the back, along with a small amount of X-ray dye, which will allow the position of the needle to be seen at all times. Then, a small amount of polymethyl methacrylate (PMMA), an orthopedic cement that becomes solid after a few minutes, gets pushed through the needle into the vertebral body. It fills the fractured vertebra and sustains the body weight after the injection for a few hours. Each vertebral body is injected on both the right and left sides, just off the midline of the back. To reduce the risk of infection, the cement is sometimes mixed with an antibiotic, as well as a powder containing barium or tantalum that allows

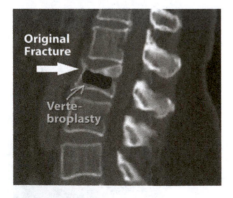

Figure 30.5 Vertebroplasty

it to be seen on the X-ray. Within a few hours, patients are up and moving around. And most go home the same day (see Figure 30.5).

Spinal fusion surgery. This procedure is used primarily to fuse or immobilize two or more vertebrae and eliminate the pain caused by any abnormal motion of the vertebrae. Supplementary bone tissue, either from the patient (autograft) or a donor (allograft), is used in conjunction with the body's natural bone-growth (osteoblastic) processes to fuse the vertebrae.

These two procedures may greatly help you reduce pain and improve your spine's stability and flexibility. However, these procedures may not solve all your problems. You may sometimes feel a great deal of pain after the procedures, and it will be necessary to have acupuncture treatments in order to reduce the pain.

TREATMENTS FOR SPINAL COMPRESSION FRACTURE IN TRADITIONAL CHINESE MEDICINE

Acupuncture

Hua Tuo Jia Ji points are sets of specially designed points used to treat spinal disease. The tender points around the spine are the ones to be treated and the needles are inserted into the disc about 0.5 inch deep, with a total of nine needles inserted into these tender points and the adjacent area.

I also selected these points: Sheng Shu, Qi Hai Shu, Chi Bian, Huan Tiao, Yang Ling Quan, Fei Yang, Ju Liao, Jue Gu, and Cheng Fu (see Table 30.1 and Figures 30.6 and 30.7).

BETTY'S TREATMENT

Betty first underwent physical therapy twice a week for four weeks in another physical therapy facility. She went through many forward-bending and backward-extension exercises, but this physical therapy caused her to feel more pain in the lower back. When I did another CT

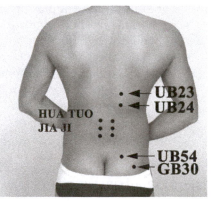

Figure 30.6

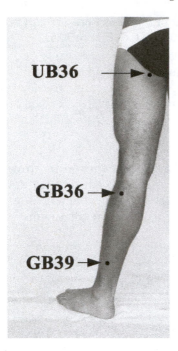

scan, I discovered that her low back compression fracture was worse than it had been on the first CT scan. I immediately directed her to stop doing the forward-bending exercise because it was causing more compression fractures.

She was referred to interventional radiology for vertebroplasty, and she felt much better after the surgery. However, two months after this surgery, she again complained of low back pain and returned to me for treatment. I gave her acupuncture treatments twice a week for four weeks and simultaneously started her on physical therapy twice a week for four more weeks. (Fosamax was also prescribed for long-term use.) After about six weeks of treatment, Betty's pain had subsided a great deal, and she became much more flexible.

Figure 30.7

TIPS FOR PEOPLE WITH SPINAL COMPRESSION FRACTURES

- You need to give up the forward-bending exercise from the low back, and try to avoid all forward-bending postures in general. For example, do not pick up any heavy objects from the floor, and try to tie your shoes by bringing your feet up so there is no need to bend down to the floor.
- You must check your BMD (bone mineral density) measurements, using DXA devices at the spine, hip, or forearm.
- For more information about the reasons, causes, and symptoms for osteoporosis, please read my previous book, *Magic Needles: Feel Younger and Live Longer with Acupuncture* (Basic Health Publications, 2011).[2]

TIPS FOR ACUPUNCTURE PRACTITIONERS

- Acupuncture can decrease the pain, but it cannot change the shape of the compression-fractured spine.

Table 30.1

	Points	Meridian/ Number	Location	Conditions Helped
1	Hua Tuo Jia Ji	Experience Points	Along the spine, use the most painful vertebral spinal as midpoint, then locate the upper and lower spinal process and 0.5 inches on either side, you may choose two spinal process as the starting points; *see* Figure 30.6.	Specifically for local neck and low back pain, and pain along the spine
2	Sheng Shu	UB 23	1.5 inches lateral to midline of spine at the level of the lower border of the spinous process of the 2nd lumbar vertebra	Nocturnal emissions, impotence, bedwetting, irregular menstruation, vaginal discharge, low back pain, weakness of the knee, blurring of vision, dizziness, tinnitus, deafness, swelling, asthma, diarrhea
3	Qi Hai Shu	UB 24	1.5 inches lateral to midline of spine at the level of the lower border of the spinous process of the 3rd lumbar vertebra	Low back pain, irregular menstruation, asthma
4	Zhi Bian	UB 54	Lateral to the hiatus of the sacrum, 3 inches lateral to the midline of spine	Pain in the lumbosacral region, muscular atrophy, motor impairment of the lower extremities, painful urination, swelling around external genitalia, hemorrhoids, constipation

(Continued)

Table 30.1 (*Continued*)

	Points	Meridian/Number	Location	Conditions Helped
5	Huan Tiao	GB 30	At the junction of the lateral 1/3 between the great trochanter and the hiatus of the sacrum	Pain of the lumbar region and the thigh, muscular atrophy of the lower limbs, paralysis
6	Yang Ling Quan	GB 34	In the depression anterior and inferior to the head of the fibula	Paralysis, weakness, numbness, and pain of the knee, beriberi, bitter taste in the mouth, vomiting, jaundice, infantile convulsions
7	Jue Gu (Xuan Zhong)	GB 39	3 inches above the tip of the external malleolus, in the depression between the posterior border of the fibula and the tendons of peroneus longus and brevis	Apoplexy, paralysis, pain of the neck, abdominal distension, muscular atrophy of the lower limbs, spastic pain of the leg, beriberi
8	Cheng Fu	UB 36	In the middle of the transverse gluteal fold	Pain in the lower back and gluteal region, constipation, muscular atrophy, pain, numbness, and motor impairment of the lower extremities

- Do not advise patients not to have surgery, because surgery might be the necessary treatment for the long run.
- Teach patients not to bend their low backs forward, as this will worsen the low back compression fracture. And be sure to tell them to avoid the forward-forward exercise.
- Patients should be advised to wear a lumbosacral brace to protect the low back during the acute stage of the low back pain.
- Acupuncture is not the only treatment for spinal compression fracture—an integrated treatment might get better results.

31

Hip Pain

Phillip, a moderately obese 45-year-old man, had pain in his right hip for five years. The pain was of gradual onset and sometimes radiated down through his right groin and right lateral thigh. He felt stiff and tight and had difficulty walking and climbing the stairs. In college, Phillip had been a football player, and now he runs and plays a lot of tennis. He did not pay much attention to the pain in his right hip until it intensified. It recently became worse to the extent that it disturbed his sleep and allowed him to walk only a short distance.

Phillip first consulted an orthopedic doctor, who ordered an X-ray, which showed the joint space was narrowing and there were degenerative changes—bone spurs and subchondral sclerosis.

Phillip's doctor told him this was typical osteoarthritis of the hip, and because the pain was so severe, Phillip was given a steroid injection right away. For two months he felt better, but as the effects of the shot wore off, the pain came roaring back. He returned to his orthopedic doctor, who gave him a second steroid injection and told him that he probably needed a total hip replacement. As Phillip was only aged 45, he was reluctant to have the hip replacement and therefore consulted me.

On examination, I noticed that when Phillip walked, he had a short swing of his right leg and could only bear weight on his right leg for a very short time. In checking his range of motion, there appeared to be decreased external and internal rotation of the hip and pain was elicited in this range of motion. An X-ray confirmed that Phillip had severe osteoarthritis of the right hip.

SYMPTOMS, CAUSES, AND DIAGNOSIS

Most people with hip arthritis complain of a gradual onset of pain in the groin. Some have pain on the outside of the thigh, buttocks, or upper leg.

The pain initially happens only with activity, but its frequency and intensity gradually increases to the point that the person will not feel relief, even while resting. There is usually severe pain, limpness, and stiffness, and pain in the night often wakes the person up.

There are different causes for hip osteoarthritis, but the most common cause is secondary, as from an injury.

Primary osteoarthritis is age-related osteoarthritis. With aging, the water content of the cartilage increases, and the protein makeup of the cartilage degenerates. The water content might also dry out after the cartilage gradually disappears, and eventually the cartilage begins to degenerate by flaking or forming bone spurs. In advanced cases, there is a total loss of any cartilage cushion between the bones of the joints.

Secondary osteoarthritis involves repetitive use of the worn joints over the years, such as found in runners, tennis players, mountain climbers, or martial art performers, that can irritate and inflame the cartilage, causing joint pain and swelling. Loss of the cartilage cushion causes friction between the bones, leading to pain and limitation of joint mobility. Inflammation of the cartilage can also stimulate new bone outgrowths (bone spurs, also referred to as osteophytes) to form around the joints. Osteoarthritis can occasionally develop in members of the same family, implying a hereditary (genetic) basis for this condition. Secondary causes of hip osteoarthritis include sports-related injuries, such as Phillip's (he was a marathon runner), that gradually change the alignment of the hip and eventually lead to wear and tear on the joint surfaces.

Avascular necrosis. This affects many who drink alcohol excessively and undergo steroid injections at the hip joint, or who took oral steroids for a long period of time (lupus, or organ transplant recipients, might also experience this condition). Avascular necrosis is the death of the femoral head without sepsis. It is caused by an interruption of the vascular supply to the femoral head. Phillip had two steroid injections, which may have caused a worsening of the hip osteoarthritis and possible avascular necrosis.

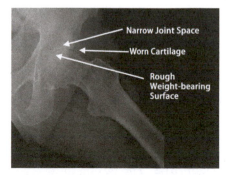

Diabetes, gout, high uric acid, obesity, surgery, and trauma are other possible causes of osteoarthritis.

Diagnosis of this condition is made by observing symptoms, **Figure 31.1** such as difficulty walking, with the person favoring the painful leg and awkwardly bending the trunk toward the affected hip. X-rays can show the classic features of hip osteoarthritis, including a narrowed space in the joint that has become hardened (see Figure 31.1).

TREATMENTS FOR HIP OSTEOARTHRITIS IN WESTERN MEDICINE

Treatment of osteoarthritis for the hip depends on the stages of the condition and the age of the patient.

Noninvasive Treatments—Early Stages

Weight Reduction

Weight reduction and the avoidance of activities that exert excessive stress on the joint cartilage can help. For Phillip, who was in this stage, it meant he needed to lose 30–40 pounds (he lost 35) and stop running and playing tennis. He was instead encouraged to peddle a stationary bicycle and swim. He rode his bike about 45 minutes a day and swam three or four times a week, and these activities, plus the weight he lost, put much less strain on his hip.

Medications

Aspirin, acetaminophen, and naproxen, anti-inflammatory lotions, diclofenac, and a Flector Patch for pain may help decrease pain.

Physical Therapy

Strengthening exercises can help, for example, doing four-way hip exercises on a mat, and working up to 30 reps for each movement (see Figures 31.2 to 31.9).

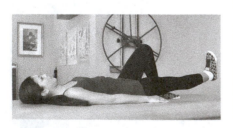

Figure 31.2   Hip flexion start

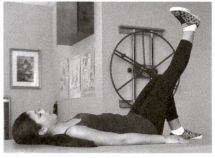

Figure 31.3   Hip flexion finish

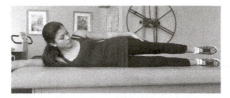

Figure 31.4 Hip abduction start

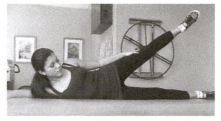

Figure 31.5 Hip abduction finish

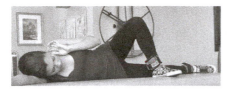

Figure 31.6 Hip adduction start
(shown with optional ankle weights)

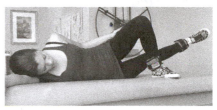

Figure 31.7 Hip adduction finish

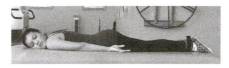

Figure 31.8 Hip extension start

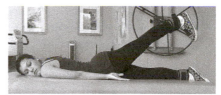

Figure 31.9 Hip extension finish

Invasive Treatments

Injections

Injecting the natural chemical, hyaluronic acid, can work by temporarily restoring the thickness of the joint fluid and allowing better joint lubrication and impact capability. Steroid injections can decrease the inflammation, thereby decreasing the pain of the joint.

Surgery—Early Stages

Arthroscopy. Arthroscopy of the hip is a minimally invasive, outpatient procedure that is relatively uncommon. The doctor may recommend it if the hip joint shows evidence of torn cartilage or loose fragments of bone or cartilage.

Osteotomy. This procedure involves cutting and realigning the bones of the hip socket and/or thighbone to decrease pressure within the joint. In some people, this may delay the need for replacement surgery by 10–20 years. Candidates for osteotomy include younger people with early arthritis, particularly those with an abnormally shallow hip socket (dysplasia).

Surgery—The Late Stages

In the late stage of hip osteoarthritis, surgery can help. Following the progress of osteoarthritis of the hip, when there is pain even at rest and difficulty walking upstairs, the use of a cane is recommended, as is a consult with a surgeon about replacing of the hip joint. A total hip replacement can bring dramatic pain relief and improved function and is now performed almost routinely.

The following are the surgical options for hip replacement.

Hemiarthroplasty. As its name implies, this is half of an arthroplasty. This procedure is usually performed as a treatment for a hip fracture. The femoral head, due to irreparable damage to the blood supply, is replaced, yet the acetabulum (socket) is in good condition and not in need of a prosthetic cup implant.

The fractured femoral head is removed; a corresponding head implant is inserted into the remained femur bone canal, and reamed to accommodate a prosthetic stem. These parts are either cemented into place or press-fit to stimulate bone growth into the prosthesis. It is a very stable combination and allows the typical older patient to reduce the risks of other medical complications (see Figure 31.10).

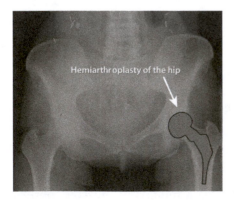

Hemiarthroplasty of the hip

Figure 31.10

Traditional total hip replacement. This surgery involves making a 10- to 12-inch incision on the side of the hip in order to dislocate the hip joint.

Once the joint has been opened up and the joint surfaces exposed, the femur, the ball at the top of the

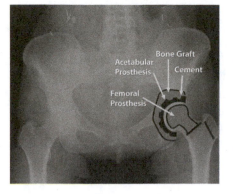

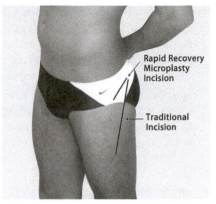

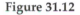

Figure 31.11 Traditional hip
replacement

Figure 31.12

thigh bone, is removed. A cup-shaped implant is then pressed into the
bone of the hip socket. It may be secured with screws. A smooth plastic
bearing surface is then inserted into the implant so the joint can move
freely. Next, the femur is prepared. A metal stem is placed into the femur,
or the thigh bone, to a depth of about 6 inches. A metallic ball is then
placed on the top of the stem. The ball-and-socket joint is recreated. The
stem implant is either fixed with bone cement or is implanted without cement. Cementless implants have a rough, porous surface that allows bone
to adhere to the implant and hold it in place (see Figure 3.11).

Minimally invasive hip replacement. This surgery allows the surgeon
to perform the hip replacement through one or two smaller incisions. Candidates for minimal incision procedures are typically thin,
young, healthy individuals. The artificial implants used for the minimally invasive hip replacement procedures are the same as those
used for traditional hip replacement. You should consult your orthopedic doctor about the possibility of this particular procedure. Its
benefits are less pain, shorter hospital stay, better cosmetic outcome,
and faster rehabilitation (see Figure 3.12).

TREATMENTS FOR HIP OSTEOARTHRITIS IN
TRADITIONAL CHINESE MEDICINE

According to traditional Chinese medicine, there are two types of hip
arthritis.

Cold stasis. The typical symptoms of this type are hip pain when
the weather gets cold, windy, or rainy. I have regularly heard my

patients tell me "I do not need the weatherman, I know when it will be rainy or snowy." This is because the patients' defensive system is not strong enough, and weather changes make the skin and joints sensitive, allowing the invasive pathogens to get into the joints more easily and make the joints stiff and painful.

Hot stasis. The typical symptoms are swelling, heat, and pain in the joints, accompanied by low fever, reddened skin, and a painful touch at the joints. Additional symptoms include thirst, annoyance, depression, constipation, hot urination, dry skin, and wasted muscle.

Acupuncture

Acupuncture must be combined with noninvasive treatments to get better results. As with other treatments, acupuncture cannot prevent the arthritis from developing further, but acupuncture can, however, dramatically decrease the arthritis pain, decrease the swelling and inflammation, and effectively delay the surgical procedure.

The main acupuncture points are GB 30 Huan Tiao, GB 34 Yang Ling Quan, and Arshi at the hip joint. The local Arshi points (tender points) at the hip joints are probably the most important points to be used for the hip pain treatment. I cannot emphasize more the importance of the local Arshi points for the hip pain treatment.

The specific points for cold stasis are GB 20 Feng Chi, UB 18 Ge Shu, Sp 10 Xue Hai, Liv 3 Tai Chong, UB 23 Sheng Shu, and Ren 4 Guan Yuan.

Table 31.1

	Points	Meridian/ Number	Location	Conditions Helped
1	Huan Tiao	GB 30	At the junction of the lateral 1/3 between the great trochanter and the hiatus of the sacrum	Pain of the lumbar region and the thigh, muscular atrophy of the lower limbs, paralysis
2	Yang Ling Quan	GB 34	In the depression anterior and inferior to the head of the fibula	Paralysis, weakness, numbness, and pain of the knee, beriberi, bitter taste in the mouth, vomiting, jaundice, infantile convulsions

(Continued)

Table 31.1   *(Continued)*

	Points	Meridian/ Number	Location	Conditions Helped
3	Feng Chi	GB 20	In the depression between the upper portion of m. sternocleidomastoideus and m. trapezius, on the same level with Fengfu (Du 16)	Headaches, vertigo, insomnia, pain and stiffness of the neck, blurred vision, glaucoma, red and painful eyes, tinnitus, convulsions, epilepsy, infantile convulsions, febrile diseases, common cold, nasal obstruction
4	Ge Shu	UB 18	1.5 inches lateral to the midline, at the level of the lower border of the spinous process of the 9th thoracic vertebra	Jaundice, redness of the eye, blurring of vision, night blindness, mental disorders, epilepsy, back pain, spitting of blood, nosebleed
5	Xue Hai	Sp 10	When the knee is flexed, 2 inches above the medial edge of the patella	Irregular menstruation, uterine bleeding, hives, eczema, sores, pain in the thigh
6	Tai Chong	Liv 3	On the dorsum of the foot, in the depression distal to the junction of the 1st and 2nd metatarsal bones	Headaches, dizziness, and vertigo, insomnia, congestion, swelling and pain of the eye, depression, infantile convulsions, facial palsy in the mouth, uterine bleeding, hernia, bedwetting, retention of urine, epilepsy, pain in the interior ankle bone
7	Sheng Shu	UB 23	1.5 inches lateral to midline of spine at the level of the lower border of the spinous process of the 2nd lumbar vertebra	Nocturnal emission, impotence, bedwetting, irregular menstruation, vaginal discharge low back pain, weakness of the knee, blurring of vision, dizziness, tinnitus, deafness, edema, asthma, diarrhea

(Continued)

Table 31.1 *(Continued)*

	Points	Meridian/ Number	Location	Conditions Helped
8	Guang Yuan	Ren 4	On the midline of the abdomen, 3 inches below the umbilicus	Lower abdominal pain, indigestion, diarrhea, prolapse of the rectum, bedwetting, nocturnal emission, frequency of urination, retention of urine, hernia, irregular menstruation, uterine bleeding, postpartum hemorrhage
9	Qi Hai	Ren 6	On the midline of the abdomen, 1.5 inches below the umbilicus	Abdominal pain, bedwetting, nocturnal emission, impotence, hernia, swelling, diarrhea, dysentery, uterine bleeding, irregular menstruation, absence of menstruation, excessive vaginal discharge, postpartum hemorrhage, constipation, weak type of cerebral vascular accident, asthma
10	San Yin Jiao	Sp 6	3 inches directly above the tip of the medial malleolus, on the posterior border of the medial aspect of the tibia; *see* Figure 31.14.	Abdominal pain, distension, diarrhea, irregular menstruation, uterine bleeding, excessive vaginal discharge, prolapse of the uterus, sterility, delayed labor, night bedwetting, impotence, bedwetting, painful urination, edema, hernia, pain in the external genitalia, muscular atrophy, motor impairment, paralysis and leg pain, headaches, dizziness, and vertigo, insomnia

(Continued)

Table 31.1 (*Continued*)

	Points	Meridian/Number	Location	Conditions Helped
11	Tai Xi	Ki 3	In the depression between the medial malleolus and tendon calcaneus, at the level of the tip of the medial malleolus; *see* Figure 31.14.	Sore throat, toothache, deafness, tinnitus, dizziness, spitting up blood, asthma, thirst, irregular menstruation, insomnia, nocturnal emission, impotence, frequency of urination, low back pain
12	Da Zhui	Du 14	Below the spinous process of the 7th cervical vertebra, approximately at the level of the shoulders	Neck pain and rigidity, malaria, febrile diseases, epilepsy, afternoon fever, cough, asthma, common cold, back stiffness

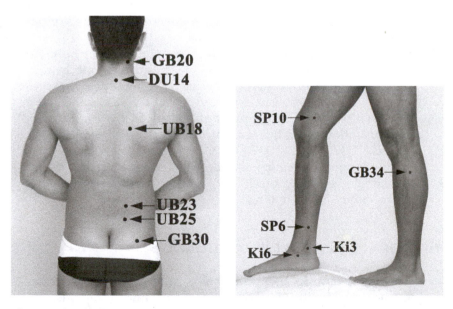

Figure 31.13

Figure 31.14

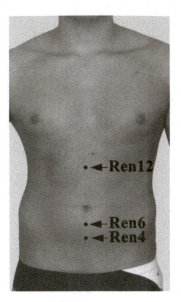

The specific points for hot stasis are Ren 6 Qi Hai, Sp 6 San Ying Jiao, Ki 3 Tai Xi, and Du 14 Da Zhui (see Figures 3.13 to 31.15 and Table 31.1).

PHILLIP'S TREATMENT

Since Phillip's goal is to delay the total hip replacement procedure as long as possible, he underwent my treatments to temporarily decrease his pain. In addition, he continues his weight-loss regime, and regularly swims and rides his stationary bike, all of which are putting off an operation for another two or three years.

Figure 31.15

TIPS FOR PEOPLE WITH HIP PAIN

- Osteoarthritis of the hip is a progressive inflammation of the hip, for which there is no cure. Acupuncture, along with other treatments, can help in delaying and decreasing the pain, but the progress of worn cartilage is unpreventable.
- For anyone in the fourth or fifth decades, a total hip replacement should be delayed as long as possible, because the mechanical joints usually last only about 15 years. If you undergo this procedure too soon, you can expect to repeat it in a decade and a half, so it would be best to put it off as long as is feasible. A second operation could increase the risks for surgery and its side effects.
- Losing weight, swimming, and peddling a stationary bicycle are the keys to helping yourself. You should not perform any sports that require a lot of running.

TIPS FOR ACUPUNCTURE PRACTITIONERS

- There are many hip diseases that also cause pain, such as greater trochanteric bursitis, piriformis syndrome, iliopsoas bursitis, tendonitis, avascular necrosis of the femoral head, and hip fractures, so it is important to properly differentiate among all the forms of hip pain.

- You must differentiate the cold type from the hot one because the treatments are different.

32

Hip Pain—Trochanteric Bursitis

Cindy is a 64-year-old woman who complained of right hip pain about six months after a fall in her garage, where she injured her right hip and immediately felt pain in it. She put an ice pack on it, took some Tylenol and Advil, and thought that would make the pain go away. It didn't. After a month, she still felt very severe pain and she had difficulty walking. She was unable to lie on her right side because of the pain, which always awakened her at night. Whenever she tried to walk, run, or lift 10 to 20 pounds of weight, the pain went straight to her right hip and made that leg feel weak. At times, it also radiated down to her knee but never went below the knee. She finally called her primary care physician, who took an X-ray of the right hip that showed no bone spur, no fracture, and no osteoarthritis. She did, however, display a slightly limited range of motion in that hip, and while the doctor was examining her, the hip swelled and felt slightly warm to the touch. The doctor told her the pain was caused by a soft-tissue injury, prescribed Naproxen, and said she would get better in about a month. But the pain got worse and worse, to the point that she was limping and leaning to the right. The pain interfered with her daily activities—driving, walking, lifting packages, lying on her right side—so she came to me for evaluation and the treatment.

Cindy is tall and moderately obese. She arrived using a cane due to the severity of the pain that prevented her from walking independently. I palpated her right hip joints, which were swollen and very tender. The pain also went along the right lateral thigh. I checked her range of motion and found it slightly limited, especially at the external rotation. I asked her to flex and externally rotate her hip by pushing outward against my hand, and this caused her excruciating pain. Her right hip joint muscle seemed weak, but I found no sensory deficit when I applied pinpricks to both legs and touched her lightly. Because the pain was so severe and debilitating, I ordered an MRI, which showed only the trochanteric bursa was swollen, tender, and had increased in size; there was no tendonitis or arthritis. Given this information, I determined that Cindy most likely had trochanteric (hip) bursitis.

SYMPTOMS, CAUSES, AND DIAGNOSIS

On the hip, there are two trochanteric bursae; one is called superficial trochanteric bursa, which is on the outside of the hip joint. The other is called deep trochanteric bursa, which is underneath the gluteus medius muscle. Hip bursitis is inflammation of the hip bursa, and those who have this condition typically complain about a lot of hip pain that very often radiates down the thigh, but the hip joint itself is not involved (see Figure 32.1).

The symptoms of trochanteric (hip) bursitis include the following.

- Hip pain that sometimes radiates to the outside of the thigh and down to the groin and knee area. The pain can worsen during such activities as running or sitting with the painful leg crossed over the opposite knee.
- Disturbed sleep due to the pain, especially when lying on the painful side.
- Swelling from the increased fluid within the bursa.
- Weakness in the affected leg that leads to limping and difficulty walking or running.
- Heat and redness in the affected bursa.

Hip bursitis is most common in middle-aged or older people and is especially prevalent among women. Among the conditions and activities that can cause it are the following.

- Contusions from falls, contact sports, and/ or by the bursal irritation resulting from friction in the iliotibial band (ITB). (The ITB goes down the outside of the leg, from the knee to the hip, and helps the leg straighten and move out to the side.)

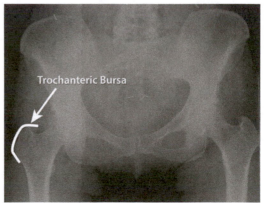

Figure 32.1

- Repetitive activity, such as stair climbing, bicycling, standing, running, or hiking for long periods of time.
- An injury, such as a fall, or lying on the painful side for long periods of time, exerting unnecessary pressure on the hip.
- Lower back pain due to arthritis, scoliosis, spondylosis, and so on.
- Previous surgery around the hip, or a total hip replacement that can irritate the bursa.
- A discrepancy in the length of the legs that changes the center of gravity and can cause irritation of the hip bursa.

Since hip bursitis is not usually related to osteoarthritis, an X-ray or an MRI will not show any hip spur, bone spur, or narrowing of the joint space. You may also not see any tendonitis around the hip joint and see only the inflamed, enlarged bursa.

The following is the differential diagnosis (a method of diagnosing a disorder that lacks unique symptoms or signs) of hip bursitis.

- Fracture of the femoral head (the highest part of the thigh bone), avascular necrosis (cellular death of bone components) of the femoral head, hip fracture, lumbosacral radiculopathy, iliopsoas tendonitis, ITB tendonitis, and internal and/or external snapping hip.

TREATMENTS FOR TROCHANTERIC (HIP) BURSITIS IN WESTERN MEDICINE

Noninvasive Treatments

Medications

Most often, a physician will prescribe anti-inflammatories, such as naproxen or Advil, but there is usually no significant improvement after taking an anti-inflammatory drug. This is because the bursitis is an acute and severe inflammation on the bursa of the hip, but many people just like to take them anyway.

Physical Therapy

A rehabilitation program involving physical therapy is very often applied and includes stretching of the iliotibial, the thigh muscle tensor fascia lata, and the external hip rotators, quadriceps, and hip flexors. Other physical therapy, including cold pads, electrical stimulation, and soft-tissue massage might be also helpful (see Figures 32.2 and 32.3).

Invasive Treatment

Corticosteroid Injections

There are many studies showing that a corticosteroid injection at the site of the inflamed bursa can be a quick, specific, and effective treatment with a prolonged benefit. Normally, the person receiving the shot should lie on the unaffected side. Then the healthcare practitioner will inject a mixture of about 40–80 mg of corticosteroid and 5 cc of 1–2 percent lidocaine into the bursa. In follow-up visits at one year and five years, about 66 percent of those injected feel much improved.

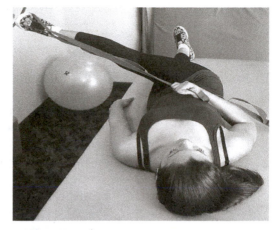

Figure 32.2

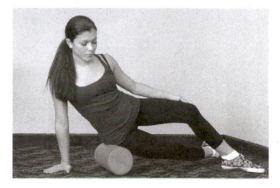

Figure 32.3

TREATMENTS FOR TROCHANTERIC (HIP) BURSITIS IN TRADITIONAL CHINESE MEDICINE

Rest and Massage

The first thing is to make sure the person rests and does not perform any repetitive activity for at least one month. During that time, treatment should include an ice massage on the hip and the ITB for about 15–20 minutes twice a day. Because the inflammation is inside the hip bursa, the fluid very often leaks out, follows along the ITB, and inflames it. That is why the pain radiates down to the thigh. Because the ITB ends around the knee, the pain will not go down beyond the knee. That makes the massage with ice a very important procedure for decreasing the inflammation and pain.

Table 32.1

	Points	Meridian/ Number	Location	Conditions Helped
1	Huan Tiao	GB 30	At the junction of the lateral 1/3 between the great trochanter and the hiatus of the sacrum	Pain of the lumbar region and the thigh, muscular atrophy of the lower limbs, paralysis
2	Feng Shi	GB 31	On the midline of the lateral aspect of the thigh, 7 inches above the transverse popliteal crease	Pain and soreness in the thigh and lumbar region, paralysis of the lower limbs, beriberi, general itching
3	Yang Ling Quan	GB 34	In the depression anterior and inferior to the head of the fibula	Paralysis, weakness, numbness, and pain of the knee, beriberi, bitter taste in the mouth, vomiting, jaundice, infantile convulsions
4	Ying Ling Quan	Sp 9	On the lower border of the medial condyle of the tibia, in the depression on the medial border of the tibia	Abdominal pain and distension, diarrhea, dysentery, abdominal swelling, jaundice, painful urination, bedwetting, urinary incontinence, pain in the external genitalia, pain in the knee
5	Xue Hai	Sp 10	When the knee is flexed, 2 inches above the medial edge of patella	Irregular menstruation, uterine bleeding, hives, eczema, skin infection, pain in the thigh
6	Tai Chong	Liv 3	On the dorsum of the foot, in the depression distal to the junction of the 1st and 2nd metatarsal bones	Headaches, dizziness and vertigo, insomnia, congestion, swelling and pain of the eye, depression, infantile convulsions, deviation of the mouth, uterine bleeding, hernia, bedwetting, retention of urine, epilepsy, ankle pain

Acupuncture

The acupuncture I usually choose is GB 30 Huan Tiao, local Arshi points (Tender points), GB 31 Feng Shi, GB 34 Yang Ling Quan, Sp 9 Ying Ling Quan, Sp 10 Xue Hai, and Liv 3 Tai Chong (see Figure 32.4 and Table 32.1).

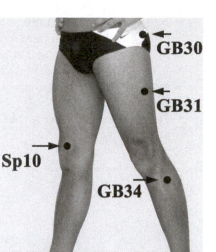

CINDY'S TREATMENT

I chose a large-diameter needle, and with electrical stimulation at the bursa and the big needle, I was able to make the swelling go down and increase the energy flow through the bursa. I repetitively stimulated the bursa, making Cindy's sensitivity to pain diminish and allowing her to tolerate more daily stimulation.

Figure 32.4

Other points, such as He Gu and Tai Chong, helped increase a large amount of endorphin secretion, and made Cindy feel less pain. She underwent my treatment for about 10 visits, and between the soft massage, the ice, and the acupuncture with electrical stimulation, she felt much better afterwards. Two months after her treatment stopped, she had a follow-up visit and I was pleased to see that her hip pain was completely gone.

TIPS FOR PEOPLE WITH TROCHANTERIC (HIP) BURSITIS

- You need to consult an orthopedic physician or a physiatrist because not all physicians can make a clear diagnosis of trochanteric hip bursitis.
- Ice massages are very important. In order to reduce the inflammation and decrease the pain, you need to use ice to massage your hip 15 minutes, twice a day.

TIPS FOR ACUPUNCTURE PRACTITIONERS

- Always ask the patient to rest and have ice massages; if you understand Chinese herbs, you can choose an anti-inflammatory Chinese herb cream to massage the patient's hip and ITB.

- If the patient's hip has an obviously severe inflammation or infection, you should not treat it, but instead refer the patient to his or her primary care physician to check if there is any infection.
- A large-diameter needle with electrical stimulation will be much more effective than a small-diameter needle without electrical stimulation.
- You may teach the patient to stretch the right ITB and hip joints in a certain way.

33

Groin Pain and Hip Tendonitis

Katie is a 55-year-old woman who loves sports and has plenty of time to play tennis, do yoga, and swim. One day, she woke up with pain in her right groin and remembered that she had jumped up to reach a high ball during a tennis competition, and this is when the pain started. It was initially on and off, and it went away in about a week. She then continued to play, but down the road she started to feel persistent pain in her groin and had difficulty standing and walking. Eventually, she was unable to climb upstairs and felt pain even when walking very slowly and getting in or out of a car. She felt better only if she rested, sitting or lying on the bed. As soon as she tried any activities, she felt persistent, sometimes sharp, pain in her right groin area that sometimes radiated to her thigh and knee. She visited her primary care physician, who gave her naproxen, but when she did not feel any improvement, she came to me for evaluation and treatment.

In my physical examination, I had Katie walk with short steps and increased knee bending while making sure her right heel contacted the ground, and her body leaned to the right in order to ease tension and prevent an overstretch of the muscles in her right hip. In the sitting position, she was holding her right hip slightly bent and extended to ease the tension in her hip muscle group and coincidentally reduce the pain in her right groin. When I touched Katie's right frontal groin area, she immediately felt tenderness and pain, but she did not have any decreased range of motion in her right hip joint and was able to lie on her right side hip without any pain. In order to rule out right hip osteoarthritis, I ordered X-rays, and both hip joints were normal with no signs of osteoarthritis, so I determined that Katie most likely had iliopsoas tendonitis, an inflammation of the tendon or area surrounding the tendon, or hip adductor tendonitis.

SYMPTOMS, CAUSES, AND DIAGNOSIS

Tenderness and pain in the groin area are the primary symptoms of this condition. Any physical examination should completely investigate the abdominal, hip, and groin areas, and, in women, a complete check of the pelvis also should be considered.

Major causes of iliopsoas tendonitis are acute trauma and overuse resulting from repetitive flexing of the hip. Hip and pelvis injuries represent 2–5 percent of all sports injuries, and among these injuries, groin pain is the most common.

Iliopsoas tendonitis and iliopsoas bursitis are closely interrelated structurally, and due to their close proximity, if there is inflammation in one, that inevitably causes inflammation in the other. Therefore, these two conditions are essentially identical in terms of presentation and management (see Figure 33.1).

The function of the iliopsoas is hip flexion, which means bringing the upper leg, the thigh, up toward the abdomen. The hip flexors are active when you perform such activities as jogging, swimming, jumping, and sit-ups, dancing, ballet, resistance training, rowing, running (particularly uphill), track and field, soccer, and gymnastics.

The iliopsoas muscles and tendons are very vulnerable to any trauma or repetitive injuries, and especially to professional or amateur athletes. Because of their complicated anatomy, many physicians may not be aware that the injuries are very frequently seen among those who perform sports. Some physicians may order an X-ray of the hip, and if it is negative for fractures or osteoarthritis, they will inform their patients there is no problem at the hip or groin. They may, however, neglect the diagnosis of iliopsoas and/or hip adductor tendonitis because muscle strain and tendonitis do not show on X-rays.

The major differential diagnosis of iliopsoas tendonitis is hip adductor strain, which also shows the pain in the groin area, although its pain is located in the medial side of the

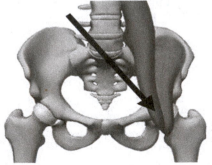

Iliopsoas Tendon
Site of Inflammation

Figure 33.1

groin area. The hip adductors are a powerful muscle group. They consist of the adductor magnus, minimus, brevis, and longus, as shown in Figure 33.2.

A hip adductor strain, or tendonitis, is a common problem among many individuals who are physically active, especially in competitive sports. Similar to iliopsoas tendonitis, the sports that most commonly put athletes at risk are American football, soccer, hockey, basketball, tennis, figure skating, baseball, horseback riding, karate, and softball.

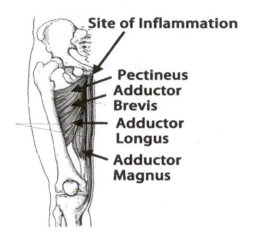

Figure 33.2

Hip adductor injuries usually occur when there is a forced push-off (side-to-side motion). Strong forces occur in the adductor tendons when the athlete must shift direction suddenly in the opposite direction. As a result, the adductor muscles contract to generate opposing forces.

The person suspected of having iliopsoas and/or hip adductor strain/tendonitis can be correctly diagnosed after a careful history has been taken and a physical examination has been performed.

These are the key points to consider include the following.

- *Get a history of the injury:* Most people have a history of injury.
- *Palpation of the tenderness:* The pain at the lateral groin is usually iliopsoas tendonitis; at the medial groin, it is the adductor tendonitis.
- Resistant flexion pain when bending the hip is iliopsoas tendonitis; with adduction of the hip, it is adductor tendonitis.
- X-rays should be used to rule out hip fracture and osteoarthritis.
- An MRI might be used in some difficult cases, but it is not usually necessary.
- Muscle strains are graded according to their severity.

    - Grade 1. Stretching with some microtearing of muscle fibers. Recovery is two weeks.
    - Grade 2. Partial tearing of muscle fibers. Recovery is one to two months.
    - Grade 3. Complete tearing (rupture) of muscle fibers. Recovery is three months.

TREATMENTS FOR GROIN PAIN AND HIP TENDONITIS IN WESTERN MEDICINE

Noninvasive Treatments

Rehabilitation Program

The initial management of an adductor and flexor injury should include protection, rest, ice, compression, and elevation (PRICE). Painful activities should be avoided. To relieve pain if there is a severe injury, the use of crutches may be indicated for the first few days.

These are the principal guidelines for this condition.

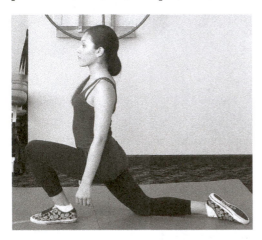

Figure 33.3

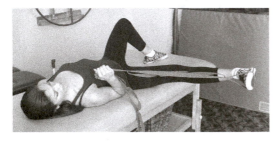

Figure 33.4

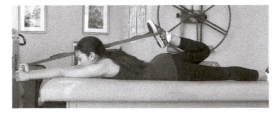

Figure 33.5

- Stop the sport right away, then apply ice to the groin area, apply elastic compression stock to the groin area, or wrap the area with an elastic band; perform a gentle stretch of the adductor and flexor muscles for one minute on each leg, up to four to six times a day, and strengthen the opposite muscles groups, such as hip extenders, or glutes (see Figures 33.3 to 33.8).

Invasive Treatment

Injections

If steroids are injected at the right place in the groin area, along the tendons of the iliopsoas, they will

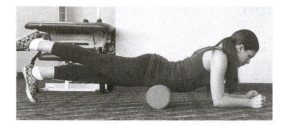

Figure 33.6

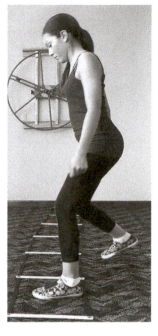

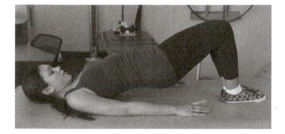

Figure 33.7   **Figure 33.8**

greatly and promptly reduce the pain and improve ADL—activities of daily living.

TREATMENTS FOR GROIN PAIN AND HIP TENDONITIS IN TRADITIONAL CHINESE MEDICINE

Acupuncture

The acupuncture points I usually choose are Sp 12 Chong Men, Sp 13 Fu She, GB 27 Wu Shu, GB 28 Wei Dao, Arshi, GB 34 Yang Ling Quan, Sp 9 Ying Ling Quan, Sp 10 Xue Hai, and Liv 3 Tai Chong (see Table 33.1 and Figures 33.9 and 33.10).

KATIE'S TREATMENT

I advised Katie to stop swimming, tennis, and yoga, and gave her about 10 sessions of acupuncture followed by massages. After these treatments, her pain was greatly relieved and she was able to walk normally and resume her active physical life.

Table 33.1

	Points	Meridian/ Number	Location	Conditions Helped
1	Chong Men	Sp 12	Superior to the lateral end of inguinal groove, on the lateral side of the femoral artery, at the level of the upper border of symphysis pubis	Abdominal pain, hernia, painful urination, local groin pain
2	Fu She	Sp 13	0.7 inches latero-superior to Chong Men, 4 inches lateral to the midline of the body	Lower abdominal pain, hernia, local groin pain
3	Wu Shu	GB 27	In the lateral side of the abdomen, anterior to the superior iliac spine, 3 inches below the level of the umbilicus	Vaginal discharge, lower abdominal pain, lumbar pain, hernia, constipation, local groin pain
4	Wei Dao	GB 28	Anterior and inferior to the anterior superior iliac spine, 0.5 inches anterior and inferior to Wu Shu, GB 27	Vaginal discharge, lower abdominal pain, hernia, prolapse of uterus, local groin pain
5	Yang Ling Quan	GB 34	In the depression anterior and inferior to the head of the fibula	Paralysis, weakness, numbness, and pain of the knee, beriberi, bitter taste in the mouth, vomiting, jaundice, infantile convulsions

(*Continued*)

Table 33.1 (*Continued*)

	Points	Meridian/ Number	Location	Conditions Helped
6	Ying Ling Quan	Sp 9	On the lower border of the medial condyle of the tibia, in the depression on the medial border of the tibia	Abdominal pain and distension, diarrhea, dysentery, edema, jaundice, painful urination, bedwetting, urinary incontinence, pain in the external genitalia, pain in the knee
7	Xue Hai	Sp 10	When the knee is flexed, 2 inches above the medial edge of patella	Irregular menstruation, uterine bleeding, lack of menstruation, hives, eczema, skin disorder, thigh pain
8	Tai Chong	Liv 3	On the dorsum of the foot, in the depression distal to the junction of the 1st and 2nd metatarsal bones	Headaches, dizziness and vertigo, insomnia, congestion, swelling and pain of the eye, depression, infantile convulsions, deviation of the mouth, uterine bleeding, hernia, bedwetting, urinary retention, epilepsy, ankle pain

TIPS FOR PEOPLE WITH GROIN PAIN AND HIP TENDONITIS

- Take a rest—stop all lower-extremity exercise for at least a month.
- Put ice on the groin area for about 20 minutes, twice a day.
- Following the above, get a deep massage for 15 minutes a day.
- If the pain is too severe, consider getting steroid injections.

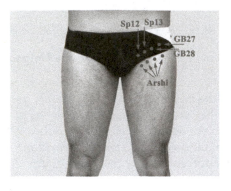

Figure 33.9

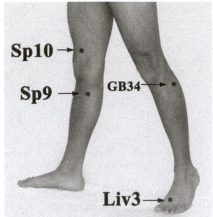

Figure 33.10

TIPS FOR ACUPUNCTURE PRACTITIONERS

- Identify the location of the injury.
- Do not use a heating pad or ultrasound.
- If the inflammation is too severe, consider steroid injections.
- All these points are a must for the treatment.

34

Lateral Thigh Burning Sensation

Janina, a 40-year-old woman, was experiencing a tingling sensation and numbness on the outside of her right thigh for six months. The pain extended to the groin area and the buttocks. Sometimes it burned, other times it was dull, and it got worse when Janina did a lot of walking or standing. At night, pain on the lateral front of her thigh sometimes woke her up. She consulted her primary care physician, who told her she probably had a pinched nerve in her lower back, and she was given physical therapy that did not help her at all. She had an X-ray and an MRI, and they showed nothing out of the ordinary.

She was frustrated by not knowing the cause of her problem and not receiving any treatment for it, so she was referred to me for examination and treatment. I found no tenderness on the lower back or lateral side of the thigh, and no decreased range of motion of the lower back, hip, or knee. The only thing I found was slightly decreased sensation in the anterior and lateral thigh, and I concurred with Janina's regular physician that she probably had a pinched nerve called the lateral femoral cutaneous nerve (LFCN).

SYMPTOMS, CAUSES, AND DIAGNOSIS

If the LFCN is compressed (pinched), this can cause numbness, pins and needles, tingling, and sometimes a burning, sharp pain in the lateral and anterior thigh. In most people, this nerve passes through the groin to the upper thigh without any compression, but there is a condition known as meralgia paresthetica where this nerve is trapped and becomes pinched under the inguinal ligament that runs from the hip to the pubic bone (a ligament is a band of fibrous tissue that connects bone to bone, or bone to cartilage, and supports and strengthens joints). (See Figures 34.1 and 34.2.)

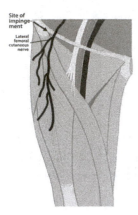

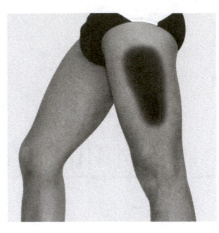

Figure 34.1 Anatomy of the lateral femoral cutaneous nerve

Figure 34.2 Sensory distribution of the lateral femoral cutaneous nerve

Common causes of this compression include tight clothing, obesity, pregnancy, scar tissue around the inguinal ligament, or conditions such as diabetes, alcoholism, or thyroid disorder. Biking, running, swimming, walking, or standing for a long time may aggravate the symptoms, and sitting tends to relieve them.

The diagnosis of meralgia paresthetica is based mainly on physical examination and patients' complaints, especially because laboratory studies, such as blood tests and imaging studies (MRIs and X-rays), are not very specific, though an EMG and nerve-conduction studies may be helpful in making a diagnosis.

TREATMENTS FOR LATERAL THIGH BURNING SENSATION IN WESTERN MEDICINE

Noninvasive Treatments

Lifestyle and home remedies, such as avoidance of tight clothes, weight loss, maintaining a steady low weight, and avoiding standing or walking for long periods, can be beneficial.

Medications

There are many useful medications for this condition, including tricyclic antidepressants and Neurontin.

Invasive Treatment

Injections

Corticosteroid injections can reduce inflammation and temporarily alleviate the pain. When the pain is severe, a local nerve block can be done at the inguinal ligament, accompanied by a combination of lidocaine and corticosteroid injections. This should temporarily relieve the symptoms for several days to weeks. Ultrasound guidance for the blockade may be beneficial in different anatomical variations.

TREATMENTS FOR LATERAL THIGH BURNING SENSATION IN TRADITIONAL CHINESE MEDICINE

Acupuncture

The acupuncture points I usually choose are Sp 12 Chong Men, Sp 13 Fu She, GB 29 Ju Liao, GB 31 Feng Shi, GB 32 Zhong Du, Arshi, GB 34 Yang Ling Quan, Sp 10 Xue Hai, and Liv 3 Tai Chong.

These insertions are combined with electrical stimulation for 30 minutes three times a week for about four weeks.

If blossom needles are used (see Figure 34.5), they should tap the front and lateral parts of the thigh, as illustrated in Figure 34.2. (See Table 34.1 and Figures 34.3 to 34.5.)

Table 34.1

	Points	Meridian/ Number	Location	Conditions Helped
1	Chong Men	Sp 12	Superior to the lateral end of inguinal groove, on the lateral side of the femoral artery, at the level of the upper border of symphysis pubis	Abdominal pain, hernia, painful urination, local groin pain
2	Fu She	Sp 13	0.7 inches latero-superior to Chong Men, 4 inches lateral to the midline of the body	Lower abdominal pain, hernia, local groin pain

(Continued)

Table 34.1 (*Continued*)

	Points	Meridian/ Number	Location	Conditions Helped
3	Ju Liao	GB 29	In the depression of the midpoint between the anterosuperior iliac spine and the great trochanter	Pain and numbness in the thigh and lumbar region, paralysis, muscular atrophy of the lower limbs
4	Feng Shi	GB 31	On the midline of the lateral aspect of the thigh, 7 inches above the transverse popliteal crease. When the patient is standing erect with the hands close to the sides, the point is where the tip of the middle finger touches	Pain and soreness in the thigh and lumbar region, paralysis of the lower limbs, beriberi, general itching
5	Zhong Du	GB 32	On the lateral aspect of the thigh, 5 inches above the transverse popliteal crease, between vastus lateralis and biceps femoris muscles	Pain and soreness of the thigh and knee, numbness and weakness of the lower limbs, paralysis
6	Yang Ling Quan	GB 34	In the depression anterior and inferior to the head of the fibula	Paralysis, weakness, numbness, and pain of the knee, beriberi, bitter taste in the mouth, vomiting, jaundice, infantile convulsions
7	Xue Hai	Sp 10	When the knee is flexed, 2 inches above the medial edge of patella	Irregular menstruation, uterine bleeding, absence of menstruation, hives, eczema, skin rash, thigh pain

(*Continued*)

Table 34.1 (*Continued*)

	Points	Meridian/ Number	Location	Conditions Helped
8	Tai Chong	Liv 3	On the dorsum of the foot, in the depression distal to the junction of the 1st and 2nd metatarsal bones	Headaches, dizziness, and vertigo, insomnia, congestion, swelling and pain of the eye, depression, infantile convulsions, deviation of the mouth, uterine bleeding, hernia, bedwetting, retention of urine, epilepsy, ankle pain

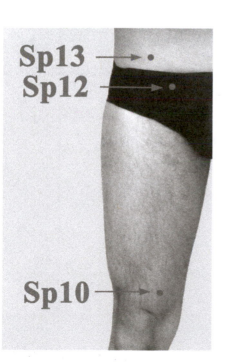

Figure 34.3

Figure 34.4

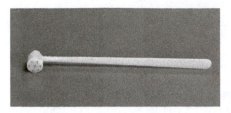

JANINA'S TREATMENT

Janina underwent treatment with both acupuncture and blossom-needle tapping and was much improved after five visits.

Figure 34.5

TIPS FOR PEOPLE WITH LATERAL THIGH BURNING SENSATION

- You need to talk to a physician about other possible diagnoses, such as lumbosacral radiculopathy, sciatica, or peripheral polyneuropathy.
- If you are wearing tight clothing, sometimes it needs to be looser.
- If you are overweight, you may have to lose weight.
- If you like biking or do other repetitive exercises, please pay attention to the inguinal area. You have to rest a while and then restart your exercise.

TIPS FOR ACUPUNCTURE PRACTITIONERS

- Make sure you have a clear diagnosis. If the patient has another illness instead of lateral femoral cutaneous neuropathy, the previously mentioned treatment will not work.
- You may have to use both body and blossom needles to treat your patients.

Knee Pain and Knee Osteoarthritis

Jonathan, a 44-year-old man, experienced knee pain on and off for two years. He played varsity football in college and after graduation took up tennis, which he played four or more times a week over the years, with no physical problems. However, when the knee pain developed, its symptoms worsened with changes in the weather. His pain also increased, even when he was only walking, and he had stiffness and swelling, with decreased range of motion when he woke up in the morning. It was difficult for Jonathan to bend or extend his knee, and when going up or downstairs, he felt as though his right knee was giving out. All of this plus severe tenderness along the joint led him to consult his primary care physician, who suspected osteoarthritis of the right knee. An X-ray was done, which showed that the cartilage in his right knee was worn out and the knee joint had a very narrow space. Jonathan was told osteoarthritis of the knee was a very serious condition and the best way to treat it would be with a total knee replacement, which he refused to do.

Jonathan then consulted me and I noted that his knee was moderately swollen. When I checked the range of motion, there was limited knee flexion (about 0–70 degrees), and when I moved the knee, I heard clicking and cracking noises, which indicated crepitation (crunching) of the right knee. I also checked the knee X-ray, which showed the knee space narrowing, and also noted some bony spurs along the tibia and fibula bones, all of which confirmed the diagnosis of knee osteoarthritis.

SYMPTOMS, CAUSES, AND DIAGNOSIS

Osteoarthritis, also known as degenerative arthritis, is the wearing out of joints during the aging process, where the older a person gets, the worse the painful arthritis symptoms become. Before age 45, osteoarthritis occurs more frequently in men. After age 55, it occurs more frequently in women.

The symptoms of knee osteoarthritis include pain around the knee, especially at the mid-joint line, difficulty walking, getting up from a sitting position, occasional swelling, and, when it is severe, obvious knee deformity.

These conditions are caused by the breakdown and eventual loss of cartilage in the knee joint—cartilage is a protein substance that serves as a cushion between the bones of the joints.

Diagnosis can be confirmed by the presence of clicking, cracking noises, which indicate crunching of the knee, a narrowing of the knee space, and bony spurs along the tibia and fibula bones.

In Figure 35.1, the knee joint on the right is a typical knee with a narrowed space indicating severe osteoarthritis, and in Figure 35.2, the left knee is a normal one with plenty of knee space.

As mentioned earlier, deterioration of articular cartilage is the main problem associated with knee osteoarthritis. The condition can be caused by a number of factors.

- *A previous knee injury.* Injuries contribute to the development of osteoarthritis. Fractures, a torn ligament, or an injury to the meniscus can affect alignment and promote wear and tear. For example, athletes who have right-knee-related injuries may try to avoid right-knee pain by leaning to the left side, but then they will be at higher risk of developing osteoarthritis in the left knee.

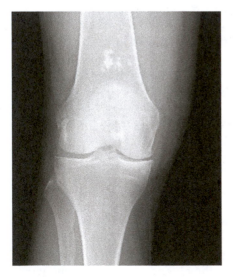

- *Repetitive strain on the knee.* Overuse of certain joints increases the risk of developing osteoarthritis. For example, marathon runners, tennis players, and football players are at increased risk for developing osteoarthritis of the knee.

- *Genetics.* Some people have an inherited defect in one of the genes responsible for making cartilage. This causes the cartilage to become defective, which leads to a more rapid deterioration of the

Figure 35.1

joints. People born with an abnormality of the spine, such as scoliosis or curvature of the spine, are more likely to develop osteoarthritis of the spine and knee because of the altered dynamic chain of the entire body.

- *Obesity*. Overweight increases the risk for osteoarthritis of the knee and hip by the addition of stress and impact on the joint surface during weight-bearing mobility. Maintaining an ideal weight or losing excess weight may help prevent osteoarthritis of the knee and hip, or it could decrease the rate of progression once the osteoarthritis is established.

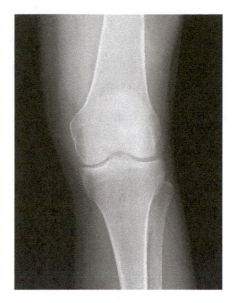

Figure 35.2

The diagnosis of knee osteoarthritis is based on a combination of following factors:

- Symptoms, including age—being older than 40, knee pain, stiffness, decreasing range of motion, muscle weakness or atrophy due to inactivity or stiffness, or a Baker's cyst (a harmless fluid collection in the back of knee).
- The location and pattern of the pain—if it is located at the midline of the knee—morning stiffness, or if the pain sometimes follows weather changes.
- Certain findings in a physical exam, such as crunching or popping in the knee joint, excess fluid in or around the knee causing swelling, or a deformity—when a malaligned knee is either bowlegged or knock-kneed.

An X-ray of a knee with osteoarthritis can show the following characteristics:

- *Joint space narrowing*. Loss of joint space is usually not uniform within the joint; the weight-bearing part of the knee joint usually wears out more. Bone-on-bone suggests there is no joint space left.

- *Development of osteophytes—bone spurs.* These protrusions of bone and cartilage typically develop as an attempt by the remaining cartilage to repair the damage, and they cause pain and limited range of motion in the affected joint.
- *Subchondral sclerosis.* Subchondral bone is the layer of bone just below the cartilage. Sclerosis means there is hardening of tissue. Subchondral sclerosis is seen on an X-ray as increased bone density and is frequently found adjacent to joint-space narrowing. The degeneration of bone that occurs in osteoarthritis causes bone to turn into a dense mass at the articular surfaces (the surfaces of a joint at which the ends of the bones meet).
- Subchondral cyst formations are fluid-filled sacs that extrude from the joint. The cysts contain thickened joint material, mostly hyaluronic acid. Traumatized subchondral bone undergoes cystic degeneration.

Sometimes blood tests will be administered to determine if you have a different type of arthritis.

If fluid has accumulated in the joints, your doctor may remove some of this fluid (in a procedure called joint aspiration) for examination under a microscope to rule out other diseases.

TREATMENTS FOR KNEE OSTEOARTHRITIS IN WESTERN MEDICINE

Noninvasive Treatments

For all knee pain, the most important thing is to divide the pain into two types.

The first type is the acute stage. In this stage the person has had a trauma or injury with acute pain, and it is necessary to use measures known as the acronym *PRICE*, which is explained below:

Protection. Use of crutches or a brace is necessary to help stabilize the joint to avoid weight bearing and prevent further damage.

Rest. Reduce or stop the activities that caused the pain, which will help reduce the pain and improve the injury.

Ice. In the acute stage, there is pain and acute inflammation. Ice will decrease this inflammation and should be applied to the injured knee three or four times a day for 20 minutes at a time. It also helps to rub the ice pack around the knee to protect the knee and decrease the pressure of the inflammation.

Compression. Use of a compression bandage and massaging the damaged tissue helps to prevent fluid buildup (edema), and hard rubbing of the knee helps to strengthen it.

Elevation. Elevating your leg with the help of gravity will facilitate the fluid return from the swelling knee to your heart, and this will decrease the knee swelling.

The second type, the post-acute stage, where there is mild to moderate knee pain, can be helped in several ways.

Anti-Inflammatory Medication

Nonsteroidal anti-inflammatory medications, such as aspirin, naproxen, and ibuprofen, help decrease the inflammation and pain.

Physical Therapy

Proper exercises will strengthen the muscles around the knee and help regain stability in the knee. A foam roller, handheld marathon massage stick, or other types of soft-issue work will assist in loosening adhesions and imbalances that can put greater stress on the joints of the knee and limit a full range of motion of the muscles (see Figure 35.3).

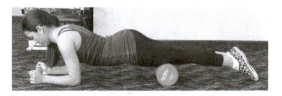

Figure 35.3

The muscles of the hip and knee must be strengthened with exercises that place less stress on the joint. These include non-weight-bearing (NWB) exercises—four-way hip exercises on a mat will strengthen the muscles surrounding the hip and knee. These should be progressed up to 30 reps each exercise on both legs.

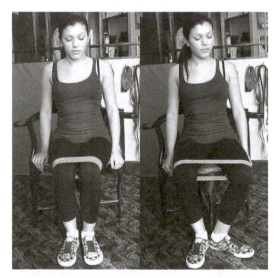

Figure 35.4

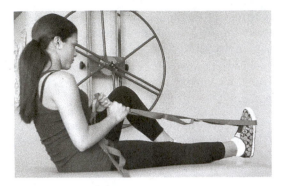

Figure 35.5

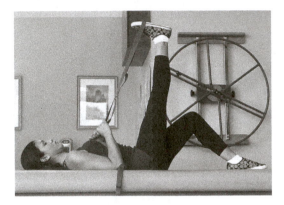

Figure 35.6

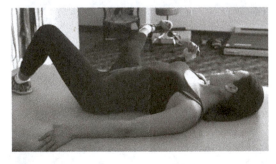

Figure 35.7

Clamshells are NWB and can be performed in a seated position or lying on your side to strengthen the muscles of the outer and inner thigh. (See Figure 35.4.)

Utilizing a stretch-out strap routine after the strengthening exercises will improve mobility in the muscles. Each stretch should be held from 30 to 60 seconds and repeated on both legs. This routine flows easily from one move to another and is NWB, so less stress is placed on the knee joint compared to having these exercises performed while standing. (See Figure 35.5.)

Stretch-out strap calves. In this exercise, you place a band around the ball of the foot and pull the band back, keeping the knee straight until a strong but comfortable stretch is felt in the calves. (See Figure 35.6.)

Stretch-out strap hamstrings. Here, you lie back and lift the leg up, keeping it straight at the knee until a strong, but comfortable, stretch is felt in hamstrings. (See Figure 35.7.)

Stretch-out strap inner thigh. You bring the leg out to the side, keeping it off the ground until a strong, but comfortable, stretch is felt in the inner thigh. (See Figure 35.8.)

Stretch-out strap outer thigh. You bring the leg across your body, keeping it off the ground until a strong, but comfortable, stretch is felt in the outer thigh. (See Figure 35.9.)

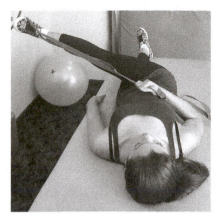

Figure 35.8

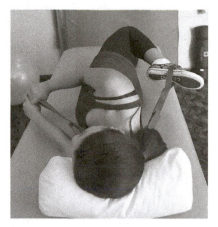

Figure 35.9

Stretch-out strap quadriceps. Lying on your stomach with the band around the ankle, pull the strap over your shoulder until a strong, but comfortable, stretch is felt in the quadriceps. (See Figure 35.9.)

When pain-free, walking is a great form of exercise. Avoid high-impact activities, such as jogging and running, and opt for walking, biking, exercising on an elliptical trainer, or swimming to improve the strength and range of motion of the leg muscles. (See Figure 35.10.)

Invasive Treatments

Corticosteroid Injections

Corticosteroid injections can quickly decrease the inflammation and pain,

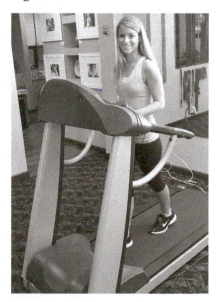

Figure 35.10

but there are many negative side effects to steroids. These include the risk of infection, water retention, and elevated blood-sugar levels, and for this reason you can't use this treatment more than three times a year.

Hyaluronic Injections

Hyaluronic acid is a naturally present substance in the human body. It is found in the highest concentrations in fluids in the eyes and joints. In osteoarthritis, the hyaluronic acid decreases, which decreases the lubrication and protection of the joint tissues of the knee, and when this was recognized, it led to the concept of injecting hyaluronic acid into knees that had osteoarthritis. One study from Canada showed that 80 percent of 458 knees injected with hylan had a positive response, and the average duration of efficacy was 8.2 months.[1]

An injection of hyaluronic acid into your knee will act as a lubricant and shock absorbent. The hyaluronic acid used as medicine is extracted from rooster combs or made by bacteria in the laboratory and is similar to the gelatinous material in the tissue spaces and throughout the body generally.

There were no systemic reactions attributed to injections of hyaluronic acid. Most of the reported adverse reactions consisted of minor localized pain or swelling, which was almost always resolved within one to three days (Table 35.1 and Figure 35.11).

A knee joint can be injected several ways. One approach is to have the patient lie supine on the examination table with the knee flexed 60–90 degrees.

Table 35.1

When to Use Intra-Articular Hyaluronic-Acid Injections

Hyaluronic-acid injections can be used under these conditions.

- If there is significantly symptomatic osteoarthritis that has not responded adequately to standard non-pharmacological and pharmacological treatments.

- When the person cannot tolerate the treatment due to gastrointestinal problems related to anti-inflammatory medications.

- By people who are not candidates for total knee replacement or who have failed previous knee surgery, such as arthroscopic debridement, for their arthritis.

- By younger people, to delay a total knee replacement. As per current studies, after a total knee replacement, the metal knee joint may last 10–15 years. For this reason, people are usually encouraged not to have a total knee replacement until age 65 or above, to avoid having to undergo two of these surgeries in their lifetime. To delay the surgery for a while, injecting hyaluronic acid into the knee joints could decrease the person's pain.

In this position, the knee gap can be opened in its maximum, it is easier to palpate, and the needle can be inserted more accurately.

The injection technique for hyaluronic-acid injections consists of Hyalgan supplied in 2-ml prefilled syringes. The recommended schedule is one injection per week for five weeks. After a hiatus of six months, Hyalgan injections can be repeated, if necessary.

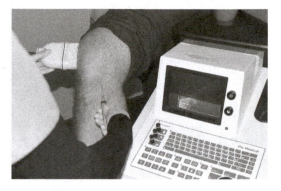

Figure 35.11

In my office, I routinely use ultrasound imaging to guide the knee injection. With this method, the injection is much more accurate and much less painful. If you would like to undergo this treatment, an ultrasound-guided injection might give you a better result.

Surgery

There are two types of surgery used for this condition.

Arthroscopic surgery will repair a torn meniscus, ligament, and tendon.

A total knee replacement is usually performed on people aged 65 and older because the artificial joint usually lasts only 10 to 15 years. If the replacement is performed too early, the person might have to undergo another one at a later time.

TREATMENTS FOR KNEE OSTEOARTHRITIS IN TRADITIONAL CHINESE MEDICINE

In TCM, there are two major types of knee osteoarthritis.

Wind hot. The knee is moderately swollen, warm, or hot with severe tenderness.

Wind cold. The knee is very stiff and feels cold and heavy. The pain is mild to moderate and is worse in the morning. There is difficulty moving and getting in or out of a car.

Acupuncture

TCM has a long history of using acupuncture to treat knee arthritis. In Western countries, acupuncture treatment of knee osteoarthritis has been intensively studied. The School of Nursing and the Center for the Study of Complementary and Alternative Therapies, University of Virginia Health System at the University of Virginia, collected 10 trials representing 1,456 participants who met the inclusion criteria and were analyzed. These studies provide evidence that acupuncture is an effective treatment for the pain and physical dysfunction associated with osteoarthritis of the knee.[2]

I choose the following acupuncture points for both types: St 35 Du Bi, Nei Xi Yan, Sp10 Xue Hai, St34 Liang Qiu, He Ding, and UB40 Wei Zhong.

For wind hot, I add Sp9 Ying Ling Quan and UB39 Wei Yang, and for wind cold, I add GB34 Yang Ling Quan and St36 Zhu San Li (see Table 35.2 and Figures 35.12 to 35.14).

Table 35.2

	Points	Meridian/ Number	Location	Conditions Helped
1	Du Bi	Stomach 35	When the knee is flexed, the point is at the lower border of the patella, in the depression lateral to the patellar ligament.	Pain, numbness, and motor impairment of the knee, beriberi
2	Nei Xi Yan	Extraordi- nary Point	When the knee is flexed, the point is at the lower border of the patella, in the depression medial to the patellar ligament.	Knee pain, weakness of the lower extremi- ties
3	Xue Hai	Sp 10	When the knee is flexed, the point is 2 inches above the me- dial edge of patella.	Irregular menstrua- tion, uterine bleeding, hives, eczema, skin disease, pain in the thigh

(Continued)

Table 35.2 *(Continued)*

	Points	Meridian/ Number	Location	Conditions Helped
4	Liang Qiu	Stomach 34	When the knee is flexed, the point is 2 inches above the laterosuperior border of the patella.	Pain and numbness of the knee, gastric pain, breast inflammation, motor impairment of the lower extremities
5	He Ding	Extraordi- nary Point	In the depression of the midpoint of the superior patellar border	Knee pain, weakness of the foot and leg, paralysis
6	Wei Zhong	UB 40	Midpoint of the transverse crease of the popliteal fossa, between the tendons of biceps femoris and semitendinosus	Low back pain, motor impairment of the hip joint, muscular atrophy, pain, numbness, in leg, hemiplegia, abdominal pain, vomiting, diarrhea, skin disease
7	Ying Ling Quan	Sp 9	On the lower border of the medial condyle of the tibia, in the depression on the medial border of the tibia	Abdominal pain and distension, diarrhea, dysentery, abdominal swelling, jaundice, difficulty in urinating, bedwetting, urinary incontinence, pain in the external genitalia, pain in the knee
8	Wei Yang	UB 39	Lateral to UB 40, on the medial border of the tendon of biceps femoris	Stiffness and pain of the lower back, distension and fullness of the lower abdomen, edema, painful urination, leg and foot cramps
9	Yang Ling Quan	GB 34	In the depression anterior and inferior to the head of the fibula	Paralysis, weakness, numbness, and pain of the knee, beriberi, bitter taste in the mouth, vomiting, jaundice, infantile convulsions

(Continued)

Table 35.2   (*Continued*)

	Points	Meridian/ Number	Location	Conditions Helped
10	Zu San Li	Stomach 36	3 inches below St. 35 Du Bi, one finger below the anterior crest of the tibia, in the muscle of tibialis anterior	Gastric pain, vomiting, hiccups, abdominal distension, stomach rumbling, diarrhea, dysentery, constipation, inflammation in the breast, intestinal inflammation, aching of the knee joint and leg, beriberi, swelling, cough, asthma, emaciation due to general deficiency, indigestion, dizziness, insomnia

JONATHAN'S TREATMENT

Jonathan underwent treatment with acupuncture and after five sessions his acute pain subsided and the swollen knee returned to normal. After the above acupuncture treatment, I injected Hyalgan into his knee once a week for five weeks. After these treatments, Jonathan reported that his knee pain had greatly subsided, and for almost a year, he was completely pain-free.

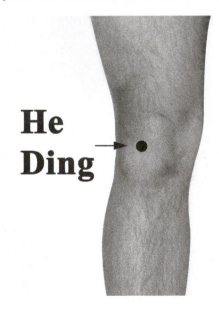

He Ding

Figure 35.12

TIPS FOR PEOPLE WITH KNEE OSTEOARTHRITIS

- Acupuncture and all other treatments besides surgery would buy you time if you have severe knee osteoarthritis. As mentioned earlier, you should have your total knee replacement as late as possible. Since the mechanical knee joint lasts only 10–15 years, you would not be happy to have two total knee replacements.

- If you have mild to moderate knee osteoarthritis, acupuncture should be your first choice because of its effectiveness and lack of any negative side effects.
- If you would like to consider Hyalgan or another hyaluronic acid injection, you should ask your physician if they use ultrasound-guided injections and if they will inject your knee once a week for at least three weeks. I prefer to inject once a week for five weeks, which would guarantee you have enough hyaluronic acid injected in your knee.

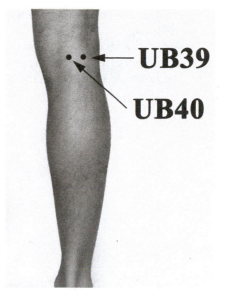

Figure 35.13

TIPS FOR ACUPUNCTURE PRACTITIONERS

- In the acute stage of any knee pain, the patient should be treated by old-fashioned methods: protection, rest, ice, compression, and elevation (PRICE).
- If an acute ligament or meniscus injury is suspected, the patient should be referred to an orthopedic or rehabilitation physician and have an MRI of the knee.
- A recent study by the National Institutes of Health showed

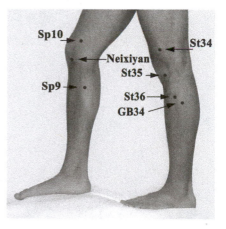

Figure 35.14

that acupuncture can significantly decrease the pain of knee osteo-arthritis.

- After the acute phase subsides, acupuncture with moxa is extremely effective for wind cold type. Acupuncture with ice on the knee is a very useful method for wind hot type.

36

Knee Pain—Meniscus Tear

Robert is a 45-year-old man who loves sports, especially skiing, snowboarding, and tennis. He came to me one day, complaining of an on-and-off pain in his right knee for about a week. He had been skiing the week before, he said, and while he was accelerating downhill and trying to make a sudden left turn, he fell in the snow and immediately felt pain in the middle of his right knee. He did manage to walk down the slope afterward, and when he arrived at the bottom, the first thing he did was put ice on the right knee. The knee had mild swelling, but as it was not so painful, he thought it would gradually subside and he wouldn't need to see a doctor. Not the case, however. Two days before he came to see me, the pain in his right knee started getting worse—he had difficulty bending that knee, and it sometimes locked in certain positions. He took Tylenol and Advil, but when they did nothing to help the pain, he came to me for evaluation and treatment. Based on his history, especially the fact that he twisted this knee during skiing, I suspected he might have either a knee sprain or a meniscus tear.

By physical examination, including the Apley's grind test (see Figure 36.5) that was positive, and the medial collateral ligament test (see Figure 36.4) that showed a vague positive, so it was medically necessary to have an X-ray and an MRI of the right knee. The X-ray of Robert's right knee showed no narrow space or osteophytes (bone spurs), which prompted me to go ahead and order an MRI. It showed what I suspected—a meniscus tear in the middle of the right knee.

SYMPTOMS, CAUSES, AND DIAGNOSIS

The definition of a knee sprain is that you have injured one of the four major ligaments around the knee joint. The most common symptoms of a knee sprain are pain, swelling, and sometimes a popping sound in the knee. Among the four ligaments, the most common form of injury is to the ACL,

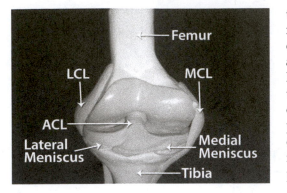

Figure 36.1

the anterior cruciate ligament. This ligament is located at the front of the knee and it prevents your lower leg, the tibia, from sliding too far forward. The ACL is critical to knee stability, and people who injure it often complain of their knee giving out. If you have a complete or partial tear of the ACL, or have frontal knee pain and swelling, you have sprained your ACL (see Figure 36.1).

The posterior cruciate ligament, the PCL, is located at the back of the knee, and its function is to prevent your lower leg, the tibia (shin bone) from sliding too far backward. Along with the ACL, the PCL helps maintain the tibia in position below the femur (thigh bone). The PCL injury is called a dashboard injury, when the knee is bent and an object forcefully strikes your tibia backwards, as can happen in a car or ski accident.

The MCL, medial collateral ligaments, and the LCL, the lateral collateral ligaments, located inside of the knee, connect the end of the femur (thigh bone) with the top of the tibia. The MCL and the LCL resist any widening of the inside of the joint, or prevent the opening-up of the knee.

A forceful impact to the lateral knee usually causes the MCL injury, and one to the medial knee causes the LCL injury.

Pain and swelling of the knee are common with a knee sprain—the tears of the ACL, PCL, LCL, and MCL ligaments. When there is an accumulation of fluid around the knee immediately after it has been injured, a possible cause is severe injury to a structure in the knee. Determining which of the four ligaments has been injured depends on the location of the knee pain—for example, the pain in the median knee might be an MCL tear; in the frontal knee, it could be an ACL tear. The main difference between tearing a ligament and tearing a meniscus is that there is swelling right away after ligament injury. With a meniscus tear, the swelling usually comes in slowly after a few hours. In order to correctly identify which structure has been injured, and strategically guide the next step for the treatment, it is absolutely necessary to have an MRI.

Meniscus Tear

The meniscuses are two wedge-shaped pieces of cartilage that act as shock absorbers between your femoral and tibial bones. The one located on the medial side of the knee is called the medial meniscus; the one on the lateral side is called the lateral meniscus. They are designed to cushion the joint and keep it stable.

Meniscus injuries are associated with cutting injuries. They occur with tibial (shin bone) rotation while the knee is partially flexed during weight bearing in such sports as American football, soccer, or skiing.

The most common symptoms of meniscal tear are as follows.

- Pain, plus you may feel and hear a pop at the time of the accident.
- Stiffness and slow swelling with a decreased range of motion in the knee.
- A catching or locking of your knee.
- Tenderness of the medial joint line indicates medial meniscus damage, and pain in the lateral joint line that may mean lateral meniscus injury.

There are three types of meniscus tears. Each has its own set of symptoms, and for each, the treatments are different.

A minor tear. You may have slight pain and swelling. It does not interfere with your daily activities, but you do feel some slight pain and minimum swelling. This usually goes away in two or three weeks.

A moderate tear. This type can cause pain at the side or center of your knee. Swelling slowly gets worse over two or three days; there is limited range of motion and moderate, tolerable pain. You may walk with mild or moderate pain, but you may feel a sharp pain when you twist your knee or squat. This pain can come and go for years if the tear is not treated.

A severe tear. With this type, pieces of the torn meniscus can move into the joint space, causing severe pain and difficulty walking. Plus, the meniscus chips can make your knee catch, pop, or lock, and you may not be able to straighten it. Your knee can feel wobbly or give way without warning. Either right after the injury, or within two to three days, the knee may swell and become stiff.

Clinically, in severe cases, a single-structure injury is rarely seen. Very often there are mixed injuries of ligaments and the meniscus. The classic O'Donoghue triad (or unhappy triad) is characterized by an injury to three knee structures.

1. The anterior cruciate ligament.
2. The medial collateral ligament (or tibial collateral ligament).
3. The medial meniscus (recent studies have shown that lateral meniscus injuries are more commonly seen among athletes).

Note: It is possible you may not remember a history of knee injury because pain and slight swelling are often the only symptoms, and you may only have noticed feeling pain after you got up from a squatting position, for example.

Other Knee Injuries

There are three other knee injuries that may mimic knee ligament and meniscus tears.

> *Patellofemoral pain syndrome (PFPS).* This syndrome is characterized by pain or discomfort that seemingly originates from the contact of the posterior surface of the patella (back of the knee cap) with the femur (thigh bone). Runners, basketball players, young athletes, and women, especially those who have an increased angle of genu valgus (knock-knees), are highly at risk for PFPS. Typically, knee pain behind your kneecap is exacerbated by sports, walking, sitting for a long time, or stair climbing. Descending stairs may even be worse than ascending.
>
> *Baker's cyst.* This is an accumulation of joint fluid (synovial fluid) that forms behind the knee. A large cyst may cause some discomfort or stiffness but generally has no symptoms. There may be a painless, or painful, swelling behind the knee.
>
> *Pes anserine bursitis (often coupled with tendonitis).* This is a painful inflammatory condition affecting the pes anserine bursa (and pes anserine tendon) on the inside of your knee; typically caused by stress to the area.

Examinations to Determine Diagnoses

The following physical examinations will help differentiate among the conditions mentioned earlier:

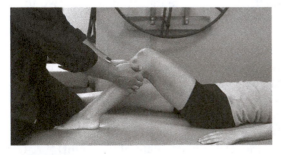

Figure 36.2

Anterior draw test. This test is used to examine an ACL injury. With the person lying supine, the knee flexed to 90 degrees, the examiner grasps the knee and pulls the lower leg forward; if an anterior motion and distinct endpoint are felt, an ACL tear can be diagnosed. (See Figure 36.2.)

Posterior draw test. This test is used to examine a PCL injury. As with the ACL test, if a posterior motion and distinct endpoint are felt, a PCL tear is indicated. (See Figure 36.3.)

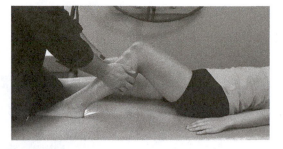

Figure 36.3

Collateral ligament test. With the person lying supine and the lower leg flattened without bending, the examiner applies force at the medial knee with one hand, and with the other hand applies an opposing

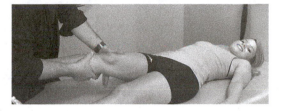

Figure 36.4

force at the ankle of the same knee. If the person feels pain at the medial knee, this indicates a possible medial collateral ligament injury. If the pain is on the lateral side, then it could indicate an LCL injury. (See Figure 36.4.)

Apley's grind test. The person lies prone with the knee flexed to 90 degrees, and the examiner presses down on the heel compressing the menisci between the femur and tibia bones. The examiner rotates the tibia while asking the person to report which portion of the knee is tender to make a diagnosis of either a medial or a lateral meniscus tear. (See Figure 36.5.)

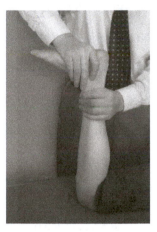

Figure 36.5

X-Rays and MRIs to Determine Diagnoses

X-rays and MRIs are the two main tests to determine meniscus tears. An X-ray can be used to determine if there is evidence of degenerative or arthritic changes to the knee joint. The MRI is helpful at actually visualizing the meniscus (see Figures 36.6a and 36.6b).

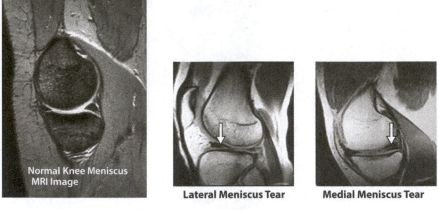

Figure 36.6a   Figure 36.6b

In an MRI, a normal knee shows smooth edges without interruption, as shown in Figure 36.6. On the other hand, when there is meniscus tear, you see the interrupted meniscus line and the non-lineated edge of the meniscus.

TREATMENTS FOR MENISCUS AND LIGAMENT TEARS IN WESTERN MEDICINE

Noninvasive Treatments

Clinically, it is difficult to differentiate meniscus tears from ligament tears. However, in the early stage, with mild to moderate cases of all the previously mentioned diagnoses, the treatment is about the same.

The acute stage. In this stage the person has had a trauma or injury with acute pain, and it is necessary to use measures known as the acronym *PRICE.*

Protection. Use of crutches or a brace is necessary to help stabilize the joint to avoid weight bearing and prevent further damage.

Rest. Reduce or stop the activities that caused the pain, which will help reduce the pain and improve the injury.

Ice. In the acute stage, there is pain and acute inflammation. Ice will decrease this inflammation and should be applied to the injured knee three or four times a day for 20 minutes at a time. It also helps to the ice pack around the knee to protect the knee and decrease the pressure of the inflammation.

Compression. Use of a compression bandage and massaging the damaged tissue helps prevent fluid buildup (edema), and hard rubbing of the knee helps strengthen it.

Elevation. Elevating your leg with the help of gravity will facilitate the fluid return from the swelling knee to your heart, and this will decrease the knee swelling.

The post-acute stage. For mild to moderate knee pain, the following can help.

Medications

Nonsteroidal anti-inflammatory medications (NSAIDs) including aspirin, naproxen, and ibuprofen, help decrease the inflammation and pain.

Physical Therapy

Proper exercises will strengthen the muscles around the knee and help it regain stability. Samples of great non-weight-bearing movements to strengthen and stretch the muscles of the leg and weight-bearing movements are described in detail in Chapter 35 concerning knee pain.

Balance training, or proprioception, is critical to retraining the stabilizing muscles of the ankle, knee, and hip. A wobble board can be used once balance in a tandem stance—one foot in front of other on a flat surface—is mastered (see Figure 36.7).

Invasive Treatments

Corticosteroid Injections

Corticosteroid injections can quickly decrease the inflammation and pain, but there are many negative side effects to steroids. These include the risk of infection, water retention, and elevated blood-sugar levels, and for this reason you can't use this treatment more than three times a year.

Surgery

Arthroscopic surgery will repair a torn meniscus, ligament, and tendon. Techniques of meniscus repair include placed tacks or suturing the torn edges of the meniscus and/ or ligament and tendon by using

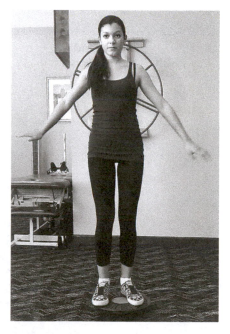

Figure 36.7

arthroscopy. Both procedures function by re-approximating the torn edges of the structures mentioned earlier to allow them to heal in their proper place and not get caught in the knee, causing the symptoms described earlier.

TREATMENTS FOR MENISCUS AND LIGAMENT TEARS IN TRADITIONAL CHINESE MEDICINE

In traditional Chinese medicine, there are two major types of knee osteoarthritis.

Wind hot. The knee is moderately swollen, warm, or hot, with severe tenderness.

Wind cold. The knee is very stiff and feels cold and heavy. The pain is mild to moderate and is worse in the morning. There is difficulty moving and getting in or out of a car.

Acupuncture

The acupuncture treatments for a knee sprain and a meniscus tear are about the same, so I choose the following acupuncture points for both types: St 35 Du Bi, Nei Xi Yan, Sp10 Xue Hai, St34 Liang Qiu, He Ding, and UB40 Wei Zhong.

Table 36.1

	Points	Meridian/ Number	Location	Conditions Helped
1	Du Bi	Stomach 35	When the knee is flexed, the point is at the lower border of the patella, in the depression lateral to the patellar ligament,	Pain, numbness, and motor impairment of the knee, beriberi
2	Nei Xi Yan	Extraordinary Point	When the knee is flexed, the point is at the lower border of the patella, in the depression medial to the patellar ligament,	Knee pain, weakness of the lower extremities

(Continued)

Table 36.1 *(Continued)*

	Points	Meridian/ Number	Location	Conditions Helped
3	Xue Hai	Sp 10	When the knee is flexed, 2 inches above the medial edge of patella,	Irregular menstruation, uterine bleeding, lack of a period, hives, eczema, skin disease, pain in the thigh
4	Liang Qiu	Stomach 34	When the knee is flexed, the point is 2 inches above the laterosuperior border of the patella,	Pain and numbness of the knee, gastric pain, inflammation in the breast, motor impairment of the lower extremities
5	He Ding	Extraordinary Point	In the depression of the midpoint of the superior patellar border	Knee pain, weakness of the foot and leg, paralysis
6	Wei Zhong	UB 40	Midpoint of the transverse crease of the popliteal fossa, between the tendons of biceps femoris and semitendinosus	Low back pain, motor impairment of the hip joint, lower extremities, contracture of the tendons at the back of the knee, muscular atrophy, pain, numbness of leg, paralysis, abdominal pain, vomiting, diarrhea, skin disease
7	Ying Ling Quan	Sp 9	On the lower border of the medial condyle of the tibia, in the depression on the medial border of the tibia	Abdominal pain and distension, diarrhea, dysentery, edema, jaundice, painful urination, bedwetting, urinary incontinence, pain in the external genitalia, pain in the knee

(Continued)

Table 36.1 (*Continued*)

	Points	Meridian/ Number	Location	Conditions Helped
8	Wei Yang	UB 39	Lateral to UB40, on the medial border of the tendon of biceps femoris	Stiffness and pain of the lower back, distension and fullness of the lower abdomen, edema, difficulty in urinating, leg and foot cramps
9	Yang Ling Quan	GB 34	In the depression anterior and inferior to the head of the fibula	Paralysis, weakness, numbness, and pain of the knee, beriberi, bitter taste in the mouth, vomiting, jaundice, infantile convulsions
10	Zu San Li	Stomach 36	3 inches below St. 35 Du Bi, one finger below the anterior crest of the tibia, in the muscle of tibialis anterior	Gastric pain, vomiting, hiccups, abdominal distension, gas in intestines, diarrhea, dysentery, constipation, breast pain, intestinal inflammation, aching of the knee joint and leg, beriberi, edema, cough, asthma, emaciation due to general deficiency, indigestion, apoplexy, hemiplegia, dizziness, insomnia

(*Continued*)

Table 36.1 (*Continued*)

	Points	Meridian/ Number	Location	Conditions Helped
11	LI 4	He Gu	On the dorsum of the hand between the 1st and 2nd metacarpal bones, approximately in the middle of the 2nd metacarpal bone on the radial side	Headaches, pain in the neck, redness swelling and pain of the eye, nosebleed, nasal obstruction, a cold, toothache, deafness, swelling of the face, sore throat, inflammation of salivary glands, lockjaw, facial paralysis, febrile diseases with sweating or lack of sweating, abdominal pain, dysentery, constipation, absence of menses, delayed labor, infantile convulsions, pain, weakness, and motor impairment of the upper limbs
12	LI 11	Qu Chi	Flex the elbow, the point is in the depression of the lateral end of the transverse cubital crease	Sore throat, toothache, redness and pain of the eye, scrofula, hives, motor impairment of the upper extremities, abdominal pain, vomiting, diarrhea, febrile disease

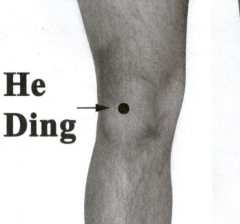

Figure 36.8   **Figure 36.9**

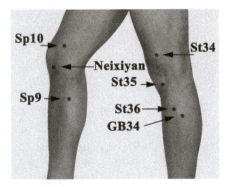

Figure 36.10

For wind hot, I add Sp9 Ying Ling Quan and UB39 Wei Yang, and for wind cold, I add GB34 Yang Ling Quan and St36 Zhu San Li (see Table 36.1 and Figures 36.8 to 36.10).

ROBERT'S TREATMENT

Robert was treated with both acupuncture and physical therapy for 12 visits. Because it was a moderate left medial meniscus tear, he did not go through arthroscopic surgery. After about two or three treatments, his knee swelling subsided, and by six visits, his pain had gradually decreased. He was discharged from my clinic after 12 visits and was given an exercise program to strengthen his quadriceps at home.

TIPS FOR PEOPLE WITH MENISCUS AND LIGAMENT TEARS

- If you have a knee injury after an accident, always apply ice to your knee, and it's also a good idea to use the PRICE procedure mentioned earlier.
- Always exercise your quadriceps muscle. This muscle group can protect your knee structures, even if you do not have a knee injury now.
- It is vital to have a clear diagnosis. If your diagnosis is a severe tear of the knee meniscus or ligament, I do not recommend conservative treatment.

TIPS FOR ACUPUNCTURE PRACTITIONERS

- Acupuncture and physical therapy can treat only mild to moderate knee sprains and meniscus tears. For severe knee sprains and meniscus tears, you have to wait until the patients have arthroscopic surgery done. You may then start acupuncture and physical therapy treatments.
- Bike and swimming exercises should be encouraged as long as the patients are out of the acute stage.
- Always encourage your patients to use ice after exercising their knees.

37

Shin Splints

George is a 16-year-old squash player who has had a personal coach training him four to five hours every day. The intensive training started when he was eight years old and made him one of the top players in the United States. One day, he complained of pain and swelling in the front of his right lower leg. When these symptoms began to occur frequently, George's coach put ice on the leg and asked him to stop training for one day. But this therapy did not make him feel any better, and he forced himself to go back to training. The dull pain was, however, getting worse, becoming constant, with the sensation of pressure. It usually felt worse at the start of his exercising and slowly subsided as the exercise continued. When George rested, he felt some relief, but the pain often returned after prolonged activity and was usually worse the next morning. When it got so bad that he had trouble jumping, running, or even walking, his mom brought him to me for evaluation and treatment.

A physical examination showed tenderness with slight redness and swelling in the front of the lower right leg and along the shin bone. The lower leg was slightly warm, and the pain spread through the entire right shin bone and felt worse at the lower half of the shin. The pain was even worse when I bent George's toes and foot downward. He walked with a limp in his right leg, and he leaned to the right, but he had no knee, hip, or low back pain. I ordered X-rays of his right leg, which showed no fractures in his right tibia and fibular bones. Based on the symptoms and the tests, my impression was that he had shin splints (medial tibial stress syndrome), a loose term describing different injuries around the lower leg.

SYMPTOMS, CAUSES, AND DIAGNOSIS

The term *shin splints* refers to pain along, or just behind, the shinbone (tibia), the large bone that goes down the front of your lower leg. There are two bones in your lower leg. The main bone is the tibia, which absorbs the impact from walking or running, and the small bone is the fibula, which attaches to and stabilizes the muscles around the tibia.

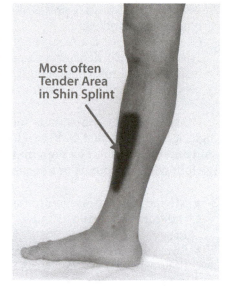

Most often Tender Area in Shin Splint

Figure 37.1

The lower leg is divided into three fascial compartments—anterior, lateral, and posterior—by three membranes, the anterior and posterior intermuscular septa, and the interosseous membrane. Because the septa membranes forming the boundaries of the leg compartments are strong, any trauma to the muscles in the compartments can produce a hemorrhage, swelling, and inflammation of the muscles. With arterial bleeding, the pressure can reach levels high enough to compress the structures in these compartments, and this will cause extreme pain known as compartment syndrome. For severe cases of compartment syndrome, the only treatment is a fasciotomy, an incision of a fascial septum (a thin membrane that divides two soft masses of tissue) to relieve the pressure in the compartments involved (see Figure 37.1).

Shin splints—swelling and pain at the medial and lower leg, in other words, in the area of the lower two-thirds of the tibia—result from repetitive microtraumas of the tibialis anterior (a muscle running from the tibia to several bones in the foot) and small tears in the periosteum membrane covering the body of the tibia. Muscles in the anterior compartment swell from sudden overuse, and the edema and muscle/tendon inflammation reduce the blood flow to the muscles. Shin splints are a mild form of the anterior compartment syndrome that develops when a muscle becomes too big for the sheath that surrounds it, causing pain.

Many athletes, including long-distance runners, tennis, basketball, and football players, or dancers, have shin splints. There are two predetermined conditions, which will make many athletes prone to shin splints.

High impact and constant stress on your shin, the lower leg's muscles and bone. This is the key contributor. If you are sedentary, and you only walk a short distance with no high impact on your leg, you will not develop any symptoms of shin splints. However, if you suddenly start to exercise without warming up, or if you have any constant, high-impact pressure on your leg, it will lead to different types of shin splints.

Overpronation, or flat feet. Many people have flat feet with no arch. This anatomical deficiency changes the dynamic chain from your trunk to your hips, knees, ankles, and feet, and puts tremendous stress on your shins, with the result that you may develop shin splints.

Other causes of shin splints include inappropriate footwear, such as high-heeled shoes, that overstretch the muscles and tendons around your shin and cause pain. The high impact and changed dynamic chain make the following symptoms or diseases possible:

- Medial tibial stress syndrome. Shin splints on the inner border of the shin, with irritated and swollen muscles, often caused by overuse.
- Stress fractures. Which are tiny hairline breaks in the lower leg bones.
- Compartment syndrome. As described earlier.

To arrive at a diagnosis of shin splints, several factors are important.

Medical history. As stated, if you have a history of lower leg pain and swelling, are warm along the anterior and posterior shin bone after excessive exercise involving your leg without warming up, or if you have pronated feet, you might have the symptoms of shin splints.

X-rays. These are usually ordered to rule out stress fractures by seeing if you have a tiny hairline fracture in your tibia bone. It is not usually necessary to have an MRI for the diagnosis of shin splints.

TREATMENTS FOR SHIN SPLINTS IN WESTERN MEDICINE

Noninvasive Treatments

In mild cases, you should treat yourself as follows:

Rest. Avoid high-impact activities that cause pain, swelling, or discomfort. Try low-impact exercises, such as swimming, bicycling, or running in water.

Ice massages in the affected area. Apply ice packs wrapped in a thin towel to the affected shin for 15–20 minutes at a time, four to eight times a day for at least one to two weeks.

Elevation of your leg. Elevate your affected leg above the level of your heart while you are sitting and sleeping, especially during the night.

Anti-inflammatory drugs. Ibuprofen (Advil, Motrin, etc.), naproxen sodium (Aleve, others), or acetaminophen (Tylenol, others) can reduce pain temporarily (but watch out for negative side effects).

Wrap your shin with an elastic bandage to protect it from further swelling. You should wrap and check it periodically every few hours. If the swelling increases, or there is more pain or numbness and a tingling sensation happens, you should unwrap it right away.

Wear proper shoes. You should wear a pair of shoes with enough space for your foot type, stride, and particular sport. If necessary, you should ask your podiatry or physiatry physicians for recommendations.

Consider arch supports and appropriate shoe insoles. Arch supports and insoles can help cushion and disperse stress on your shinbones.

Physical Therapy

In moderate cases of shin splints, you may need some physical therapy. Stretches for the lower leg muscles include calf stretches. Maintaining a straight back leg will put an emphasis on the calf muscle, and a bent back leg shift will target the soleus muscle (see Figures 37.2 and 37.3). The back ankle should be held on the ground with toes pointing straight forward,

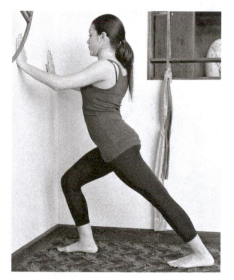

Figure 37.2

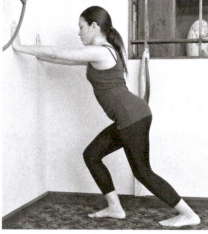

Figure 37.3

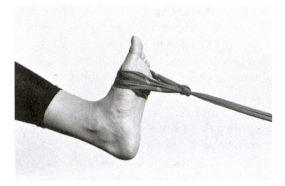

Figure 37.4

and each stretch should be held for 30–60 seconds.

Strengthening the muscles of the ankle and lower leg is important to prevent imbalances in that area. The exercises should be performed pain-free for 20–30 reps before adding resistance from a Thera-Band, as demonstrated in Figures 37.3 and 37.4. The person should build up to three sets of 10 reps for each of these exercises, which are referred to as four-way ankle exercises. The first motion is to pull the foot back toward the body as resistance is applied in the opposite direction. The next motion is to push the foot down and away from the body against resistance. The third motion is to turn the foot down and

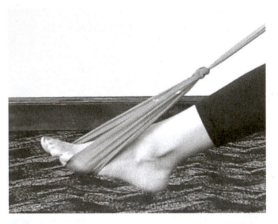

Figure 37.5

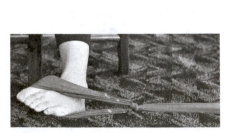

Figure 37.6

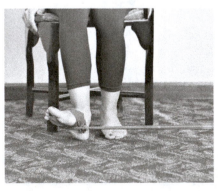

Figure 37.7

in against the Thera-Band. The final motion is to turn the foot up and out (see Figures 37.4 to 37.7).

Invasive Treatment

Surgery

As mentioned earlier, for severe cases of compartment syndrome, the only treatment is a fasciotomy, an incision of a fascial septum (a thin membrane that divides two soft masses of tissue) to relieve the pressure in the compartments concerned. Otherwise, there is no need to have surgery for simple shin splint.

TREATMENTS FOR SHIN SPLINTS IN TRADITIONAL CHINESE MEDICINE

Acupuncture

I usually choose the following acupuncture points: For both sides LI 4 He Gu, LI 11 Qu Chi. Then I choose a different group, depending on which compartments are in need of treatment.

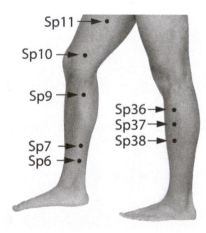

Figure 37.8

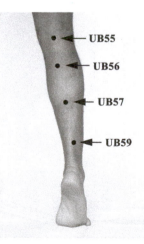

Figure 37.9

Table 37.1

	Points	Meridian/Number	Location	Conditions Helped
1	San Yin Jiao	Sp 6	3 inches directly above the tip of the medial malleolus, on the posterior border of the medial aspect of the tibia; see Figure 37.8	Abdominal pain, distension, diarrhea, irregular menstruation, uterine bleeding, prolapse of the uterus, sterility, delayed labor, night bedwetting, impotence, bedwetting, painful urination, edema, hernia, pain in the external genitalia, muscular atrophy, motor impairment, paralysis, and leg pain, headaches, dizziness and vertigo, insomnia
2	Lou Gu	Sp 7	3 inches above Sp 5 on the line joining the tip of the medial malleolus and Sp9	Abdominal distension, stomach rumbling, coldness, numbness and paralysis of the knee and leg
3	Ying Ling Quan	Sp 9	On the lower border of the medial condyle of the tibia, in the depression on the medial border of the tibia	Abdominal pain and distension, diarrhea, dysentery, edema, jaundice, difficult urination, bedwetting, incontinence of urine, pain in the external genitalia, dysmenorrheal, pain in the knee
4	Xue Hai	Sp 10	When the knee is flexed, 2 inches above the medial edge of patella	Irregular menstruation, uterine bleeding, amenorrhea, urticaria, eczema, acute skin condition, pain in the medial aspect of the thigh

5	Ji Men	6 inches above Sp 10 on the line drawn from S10 to Sp12	Painful urination, bedwetting, pain and swelling in the inguinal region, muscular atrophy, motor impairment, pain and paralysis of the lower extremities
6	Zu San Li	Stomach 36	3 inches below St. 35 Du Bi, one finger below the anterior crest of the tibia, in muscle of the tibialis anterior	Gastric pain, vomiting, hiccups, abdominal distension, rumbling stomach, diarrhea, dysentery, constipation, inflammation of the breast, inflammation of the intestines, aching of the knee joint and leg, beriberi, edema, cough, asthma, emaciation due to general deficiency, indigestion, apoplexy, paralysis, dizziness, insomnia
7	Shang Ju Xu	St 37	3 inches below St 36, one finger-breadth from the anterior crest of the tibia in the tibialis anterior	Abdominal pain and distension, rumbling stomach, diarrhea, dysentery, constipation, inflamed intestines, paralysis due to stroke, beriberi
8	Xia Ju Xu	St 39	3 inches below St 37, one finger-breadth from the anterior crest of the tibia in the muscle of tibialis anterior	Lower abdominal pain, backache referring to the testis, breast inflammation, numbness, and paralysis of the lower extremities

(*Continued*)

267

Table 37.1 (*Continued*)

	Points	Meridian/Number	Location	Conditions Helped
9	Feng Long	St 40	8 inches superior to the external malleolus, about one finger-breadth lateral to St 38	Headaches, dizziness and vertigo, cough, asthma, excessive sputum, pain in the chest, constipation, mania, epilepsy, muscular atrophy, motor impairment, pain, swelling, or paralysis of the lower extremities
10	He Yang	UB 55	2 inches directly below UB 40, between the medial and lateral heads of gastrocnemius, on the line joining B 40 and B 57	Low back pain, pain and paralysis of the lower extremities
11	Cheng Jing	UB 56	Midway between UB 55 and UB 57, in the center of the belly of gastrocnemius	Spasm of the big calf muscle, hemorrhoids, acute low back pain
12	Cheng Shan	UB 57	Directly below the belly of gastrocnemius, on the line joining UB 40 and tendo calcaneus, about 8 inches below UB 40	Low back pain, spasm of the big calf muscle, hemorrhoids, constipation, beriberi
13	Fu Yang	UB 59	3 inches directly above UB 60	Heavy sensation of the head, headaches, low back pain, redness and swelling of the external shin bone, paralysis of the lower extremities

For the anterior and lateral compartments, I choose Sp 6 San Ying Jiao, Sp 7 Lou Gu, Sp 8 Di Ji, Sp 9 Ying Ling Quan, Sp 10 Xue Hai, Sp 11 Ji Men, St 36 Zu San Li, St 37 Shang Ju Xu, and St 39 Xia Ju Xu.

For the posterior compartment, I choose UB 55 He Yang, UB 56 Cheng Jing, UB 57 Cheng Shan, and UB 59 Fu Yang (see Figures 37.8 and 37.9 and Table 37.1).

GEORGE'S TREATMENT

George was asked to stop playing squash immediately. To reduce his inflammation, he was advised to have an ice massage for two weeks on the right shin for 10 minutes four or five times a day. Acupuncture treatment was performed three times a week for four weeks, accompanied by physical therapy. After these treatments, his right shin splints were much better, and in two months he was able to return to his squash training.

TIPS FOR PEOPLE WITH SHIN SPLINTS

- If you have flat feet, please try to use a pair of arch supports, which will help you prevent shin splints from occurring.
- Warm up 15 minutes before you do any high-impact sports, such as running, tennis, jumping, or martial arts.
- After your high-impact sports, always ice massage your shin bone for 10–15 minutes, even if you only have a slight pain in your shin bone.
- Prevention is better than treatment.

TIPS FOR ACUPUNCTURE PRACTITIONERS

- Always inform your patients about the importance of self-care, such as ice massage, arch supports, and appropriate footwear for high-impact sports. If they do long-distance running, they need to get new shoes every 350 miles.
- Acupuncture treatment accompanied by 30 minutes of electrical stimulation will get the best results.
- You should not use moxibustion for patients with shin splints.
- Concerning severe compartment syndrome: If you cannot feel a pulse in the patient's feet, you must send the patient to a surgeon ASAP. The leg might be saved if the patient has a fasciotomy within a few hours.

38

Ankle Pain

Douglas is a 26-year-old football player who began experiencing right lateral ankle pain after a month of strenuous exercise. He was training for the 100-meter dash when he felt a sharp pain in his right ankle that caused him to fall. He was immediately taken to a sports medicine doctor, who found his right ankle to be moderately swollen, but because of the severe pain, the doctor immediately sent Douglas for an MRI of the right ankle. Although the MRI showed no fracture and no ankle-bone dislocation, it did show a sprained ligament of the right ankle.

Douglas was given preventive treatment known as *PRICE*.

In the acute stage, after the person has had a trauma or injury with acute pain, it is necessary to use measures known by the acronym PRICE.

Protection. Use of crutches or a brace is necessary to help stabilize the joint, avoid weight bearing, and prevent further damage.

Rest. Reduce or stop the activities that caused the pain, which will help reduce the pain and improve the injury.

Ice. In this stage, there is pain and acute inflammation. Ice will decrease this inflammation and should be applied to the injured knee three or four times a day for 20 minutes at a time. It also helps rub the ice pack around the knee to protect the knee and decrease the pressure of the inflammation.

Compression. Using a compression bandage and massaging the damaged tissue helps prevent fluid buildup (edema), and hard rubbing of the knee helps strengthen it.

Elevation. Elevating your leg with the help of gravity will facilitate the fluid return from the swelling knee to your heart, and this will decrease the knee swelling.

Although he gradually felt better, Douglas still felt pain in the right lateral ankle after a month, so he came to me for further treatment and evaluation. I noted the ankle was still slightly swollen and the lateral right side of it was very tender. His range of motion of the right ankle with his right foot bent up toward his nose was 0–30 degrees, and his foot bent down to the ground was 0–20 degrees, though with pain.

Douglas had a lateral ankle sprain, the most common form of ankle sprains, which accounts for 80 percent of the injuries of this type.

SYMPTOMS, CAUSES, AND DIAGNOSIS

There are three small ligaments in the ankle that are very easy to sprain.

Anterior talofibular ligament (ATFL). This ligament is the most common one to be injured.

Calcaneofibular ligament (CFL). This is the second most common.

Posterior talofibular ligament (PTFL). This is the last to be injured (see Figure 38.1).

All three of these ligaments function to stabilize the ankle during inversion (when the ankle gets strongly turned in—see Figure 38.2), so this is the most vulnerable position when the ankle experiences an inversion-type twist of the foot that is generally followed by pain and swelling.

The ankle pain is most often caused by injury to the ligaments, not the bones. Ankle ligaments, especially, are most commonly injured when the foot is turned inward or inverted by a force greater than the ankle ligaments can sustain.

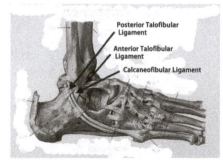

Figure 38.1

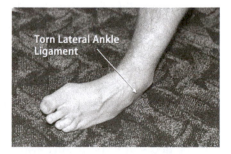

Figure 38.2

This kind of injury can happen in a number of ways.

- When the athlete lands wrong in such sports as football, basketball, or tennis. A common example is a basketball player who goes up for a rebound and comes down on top of another player's foot. This can cause the rebounder's foot to roll inward.
- In a fall, while stepping in a hole or any irregular surface.

For purposes of diagnosis, there are three grades of lateral ankle sprains.

Grade 1 is mild. This type includes a partial tear of the ATFL and intact CFL and PTFL. There is mild swelling and point tenderness, but no instability of the ankle.

Grade 2 is moderate. There is a complete tear of the ATFL and a partial tear of the CFL. The ankle is very unsteady and exhibits diffuse swelling and a bruise caused by bleeding underneath the skin.

Grade 3 is severe. There is a complete tear of both the ATFL and the CFL, causing extreme unsteadiness.

TREATMENTS FOR ANKLE PAIN IN WESTERN MEDICINE

During the acute stage, the ankle is treated with PRICE, as detailed earlier. Nonsurgical treatment can treat only grade 1 and possibly part of grade 2. Grade 3 requires surgery.

Noninvasive Treatments

Physical Therapy

A rocker boot helps promote a more natural gait while providing stability for severely sprained ankles or fractures of the foot. It is also used postoperatively. There are many types of rocker boots, but most of them feature adjustable air cells to ensure a custom snug fit to accommodate any foot. (See Figure 38.3.)

Ensuring optimal pain-free motion is necessary for a successful recovery. Strengthening the muscles of the ankle and lower leg is

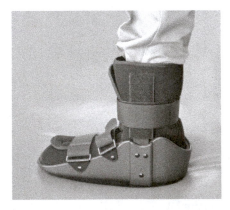

Figure 38.3   Rocker boot

important to prevent imbalances and future weakness in the ankle. Starting with active range-of-motion exercises, perform up to 30 pain-free reps of the four-way ankle movements before moving on to resistance with strengthening. (See Figures 38.4 to 38.7.)

> *Dorsiflexion.* The foot is pulled back toward the body against resistance.
>
> *Plantarflexion.* The foot is pushed down and away from the body against resistance.
>
> *Inversion.* The foot is turned down and in against resistance.
>
> *Eversion.* The foot is turned up and out against resistance.

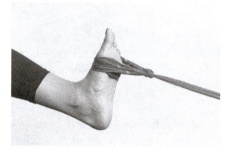

Figure 38.4 The ankle and foot dorsal flexion exercise. The foot goes up toward the knee.

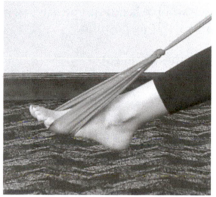

Figure 38.5 The ankle and foot plantar flexion exercise. The foot goes down toward the ground.

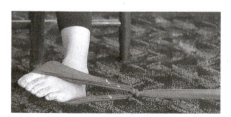

Figure 38.6 The ankle and foot inversion exercise. The foot goes inward.

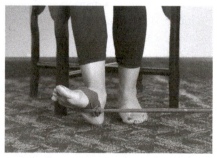

Figure 38.7 The ankle and foot eversion exercise. The foot goes outward.

These exercises are intended to continue strengthening the stabilizing muscles of the ankle and improve proprioception work on balance when standing on the ground.

Afterward, continue to progress by doing two sets of balancing with a foam pad for 30 seconds each time. (See Figure 38.8.)

This will assist in strengthening the stabilizing muscles of the ankle and help regain balance in case the ankle is injured again, as, for example, when coming down on your own ankle and twisting it. Once balance is achieved standing on a flat surface and on the foam pad, the wobble board can be used again, this time in a standing position.

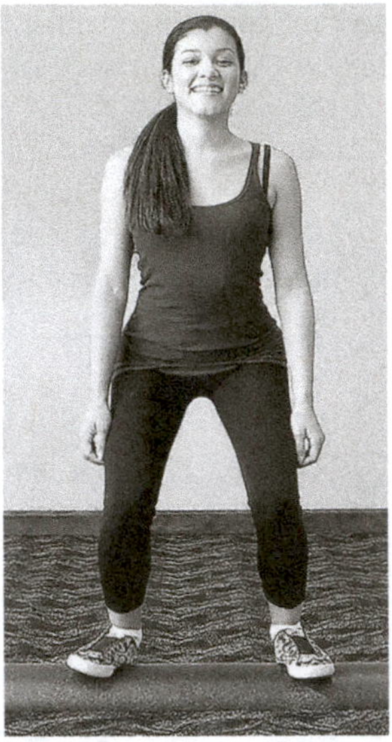

Invasive Treatment

Surgery

Figure 38.8

For grades 1 and 2, the conservative treatments as outlined here are enough. For grade 3, there may still be a reason to try a six-month rehabilitation, acupuncture, and a brace. However, if conservative treatment fails on a high-performance athlete who still has persistent ankle instability, then surgical reconstruction of torn ligaments may be considered as early as three months post-injury. Surgical treatment for ankle sprains is rare. Surgery is reserved for injuries that fail to respond to nonsurgical treatment, and for persistent instability after months of rehabilitation and nonsurgical treatment.

Surgical options include the following

Arthroscopy. A surgeon looks inside the joint to see if there are any loose fragments of bone or cartilage, or if part of the ligament is caught in the joint.

Reconstruction. A surgeon repairs the torn ligament with stitches (sutures), or uses other ligaments and/or tendons found in the foot and around the ankle to repair the damaged ligaments.

TREATMENTS FOR ANKLE PAIN IN TRADITIONAL CHINESE MEDICINE

Many people have tried everything before they come to me. They have usually had different treatments for years but still feel pain and have difficulty standing and walking. And when they walk a long distance, as during a vacation, the pain they experience is extreme. Acupuncture might well be a last resort for them.

The first thing is to make a clear diagnosis by palpating the tender points to differentiate between injuries of the three ligaments. The most commonly injured ligament is the ATFL; the second most commonly injured ligaments are the ATFL and CFL combined. You will see rarely a PTFL injury. After palpation, you can clearly understand the source of the problems and can then treat the injury appropriately.

Acupuncture

The following acupuncture points are usually selected: Sp 6 San Ying Jiao, UB 62 Sheng Mai, GB 40 Qiu Xu, UB 60 Kun Lun, PC 6 Nei Guan, and St 36 Zu San Li.

Sp 6 is the crossing point for three ying meridians; therefore, it can adjust the energy of all three meridians and smooth the blood and qi. UB 62 is located at the ATFL, so it is very important to use this for the ATFL injury. GB 41, coincidentally located at the CFL, will help UB 62, and both UB 62 and GB 41 will bring blood flow to the injured ATFL and CFL ligaments

Table 38.1

	Points	Meridian/ Number	Location	Conditions Helped
1	San Yin Jiao	Sp 6	3 inches directly above the tip of the medial malleolus, on the posterior border of the medial aspect of the tibia; *see* Figure 38.9.	Abdominal pain, diarrhea, irregular menstruation, uterine bleeding, prolapse of the uterus, sterility, delayed labor, night bedwetting, involuntary urinating, painful urination impotence, swelling, hernia, pain in the external genitalia, muscular atrophy, motor impairment, paralysis, and leg pain, headaches, dizziness, and vertigo, insomnia

(Continued)

Table 38.1   (*Continued*)

	Points	Meridian/ Number	Location	Conditions Helped
2	Shen Mai	UB 62	In the depression directly below the external malleolus	Epilepsy, mania, headaches, dizziness, insomnia, backache, aching of the leg
3	Qiu Xu	GB 40	Anterior and inferior to the external malleolus, in the depression on the lateral side of the tendon of extensor digitorum longus	Pain in the neck, vomiting, acid regurgitation, muscular atrophy of the lower limbs, pain and swelling of the external shin bone, malaria
4	Kun Lun	UB 60	In the depression between the external malleolus and Achilles tendon	Headaches, blurring of vision, neck rigidity, nosebleed, pain in the shoulder, back, and arm, swelling and heel pain, difficult labor, epilepsy
5	Nei Guan	PC 6	2 inches above the transverse crease of the wrist, between the tendons of m. palmaris longus and m. flexor radialis	Cardiac pain, palpitations, stuffy chest, stomach ache, nausea, vomiting, hiccups, mental disorders, epilepsy, insomnia, febrile diseases, irritability, malaria, contracture and pain of the elbow and arm
6	Zu San Li	St 36	3 inches below St. 35 Du Bi, one finger below the anterior crest of the tibia, in the muscle of tibialis anterior	Gastric pain, vomiting, hiccups, abdominal distension, gas, diarrhea, dysentery, constipation, inflamed intestinal tract, aching of the knee joint and leg, beriberi, edema, cough, asthma, emaciation due to general deficiency, indigestion, apoplexy, paralysis, dizziness, insomnia

to facilitate healing. PC 6 and St 36 help adjust the entire energy flow in the body (see Table 38.1 and Figure 38.9).

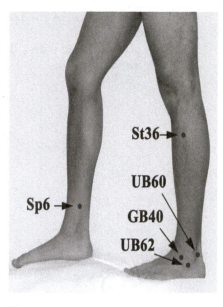

TREATMENT FOR DOUGLAS

Douglas underwent my treatment two or three times a week for about five weeks. In addition to acupuncture, he was guided to have strengthening exercise for his right ankle. I realized that acupuncture alone might take him a longer time to recover, but if acupuncture was combined with physical therapy and an ankle brace, Douglas would have much less pain and could resume his regular exercising walk sooner, which he did after five weeks of treatment. Although there is some mild tenderness, he can now sustain much longer ambulation and training without pain.

Figure 38.9

TIPS FOR PEOPLE WITH ANKLE PAIN

- For a severe grade 3 sprain, you may want to consider surgery for a solution to the problem. However, if you have a grade 1 or 2 sprain, be very cautious about having surgery. I have patients who went through many surgeries but have still had long-term pain for many years.
- Every day you should massage the three points—UB 60, UB 62, and GB 40 (see Figure 38.9)— for 5–10 minutes in both the morning and evening. If you apply anti-inflammatory cream for massages, you will get better results.

TIPS FOR ACUPUNCTURE PRACTITIONERS

- Acupuncture and physical therapy can treat only a grade 1 ankle sprain. If the sprain is grade 2 or 3, you should encourage the patient to consult an orthopedic physician.
- Acupuncture is a good treatment for long-term ankle pain, but you may need to treat the patient for a few months to get better results.

- You should encourage your patients to use an ankle brace to protect the ankle joint.
- Electrical stimulation with UB 60, UB 62, and GB 40 for 30 minutes is very important.

39

Achilles Tendon Injury

Eric is a 55-year-old man who played tennis in the past and began training for a marathon, believing he would be an excellent marathon runner. He got up around 5 A.M., ran about two hours, and then went to work. He ran a total of five or six days a week until he had a slight fall during his training. He heard a popping sound, and there was immediate swelling and a sharp pain on the back of the right ankle, which left him unable to walk. He called his primary care doctor right away and was referred to an orthopedic physician, who carefully examined him and suspected a tear in the Achilles tendon. An MRI confirmed a partial tear in the right Achilles tendon, and Eric was advised to stop his marathon training immediately. Ice was put on this tendon, and he was instructed to rest his ankle for a month and wait to see what developed. He was also told to massage the area with ice three times a day for 10 minutes each time, and was further advised that if the tendon did not heal, he might need surgery to repair it.

Two months after his accident, Eric came to see me for evaluation and treatment and reported that his right ankle was still painful and had mild swelling. He had tried ice massages and rest during this time but still felt severe pain at right back of the ankle. The orthopedic doctor had said that his Achilles tendon was healing and so it was not necessary to have surgery. In spite of this, he still felt a lot of pain and could walk only one block without pain.

In my physical examination of Eric's right ankle, I saw swelling and a tender Achilles tendon with some floating fluid inside. Additionally, he did not have a full range of motion in this ankle, leading me to believe that his problem was Achilles tendonitis.

SYMPTOMS, CAUSES, AND DIAGNOSIS

The Achilles tendon, the thickest and strongest tendon in the body, is located at back of the ankle and connects the calf muscles at the back of the lower leg to the heel bone. The leg muscles it connects to are the most powerful muscle group in the body. When these calf muscles contract, they pull the Achilles tendon upward, which pushes the foot downward and makes standing on toes, walking, running, and jumping possible. Each Achilles tendon sustains a person's entire body weight with each step. Depending on the speed, stride, terrain, and additional weight being carried or pushed, each Achilles tendon may be subject to 3–12 times a person's body weight during a sprint or push-off. One study showed that the Achilles tendon has a poor blood supply throughout its length, and this may prevent adequate tissue repair following trauma, leading to a further weakening of the tendon.[1]

Achilles tendonitis is an inflammation of the Achilles tendon, caused by microtears and repetitive off-center overloads on the tendon. There is also new evidence of Achilles tendinosis (most people in the medical field still call it Achilles tendonitis) where there is *no* inflammation in the Achilles tendon, and the cells of the Achilles tendon are disorganized, degenerated, and scarred.

Achilles tendonitis is often the result of sports-related injuries, including running, that develop from overuse, intense exercise, jumping, or any activities that strain the tendon and calf muscles. People who have Achilles tendonitis usually lack flexibility and do not warm up the Achilles tendon before their activities.

Reasons for the damage to the Achilles tendon include the following factors.

- Inflammation and degeneration cause a series of micro-ruptures and breakdowns in the collagen fibers.
- Poor nutrition. Inadequate flow of blood to the area near the insertion of the tendon.
- Mechanical. Sudden push-off with the foot in the extension position, such as landing from a jump.
- Gradual pain, with the pain worsening over time at the back of the ankle, is the most common sign of Achilles tendonitis.

Achilles tendonitis includes these signs and symptoms that can be used to diagnose the problem.

- Mild pain at the back of the ankle after running or other sports activities.

- Pain that gets worse after prolonged running, tennis, climbing stairs, jumping, or other activities. The patient experiences stiffness and has difficulty walking, especially in the morning.
- If a partial tear is involved, swelling and/or a bump might show on the Achilles tendon, and a crackling or creaking sound might be heard when touching or moving the Achilles tendon.

TREATMENTS FOR ACHILLES TENDON INJURY IN WESTERN MEDICINE

Noninvasive Treatments

1. *For acute Achilles tendonitis,* the *PRICE* treatment is recommended.

   Pressure. Apply pressure on the Achilles tendon with an ice bag for 15–30 minutes.
   Rest. Stop lower-extremity sports, such as running or biking, for at least two to four weeks. Upper-extremity exercises, such as bench presses or weight lifts, can continue.
   Ice. As noted earlier.
   Compression. Wrap an Ace bandage around the Achilles tendon.
   Elevation. To avoid fluid retention, elevate the foot as much as possible.

2. *Avoid anti-inflammatory medication.* Tylenol or Advil will not help heal the inflammation. The purpose of painkillers is to mask pain, but because you cannot feel any pain, you may further injure your Achilles tendon.

3. *Avoid steroid injections.* Injections of steroids at the Achilles tendon can cause a further rupture.

Physical Therapy

For chronic Achilles tendonitis, physical therapy is recommended. As shown in Figures 39.1 and 39.2, both the larger calf muscle, called the gastrocnemius, and the soleus, a smaller muscle deep in the calf, need to be stretched, with both a straight leg and a slightly bent leg, and each position needs to be held for one minute.

Stretches for the Achilles tendon can also be performed on a specific device called ProStretch, or off any sturdy step, and held for one minute each. (See Figures 39.3 and 39.4.)

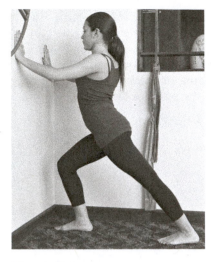

Figure 39.1

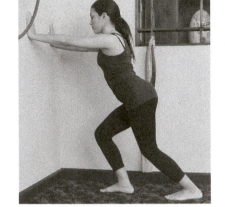

Figure 39.2

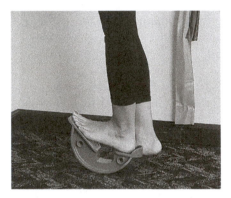

Figure 39.3

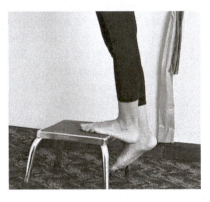

Figure 39.4

Heel Lifts and Shoe Wedges

There are many products on the market for heel lifts. The principle is to lift the heel and reduce the stress on the Achilles tendon.

You may simply put the heel lift inside your shoe or have a shoe wedge outside the shoe to help reduce the stretch of the Achilles tendon.

Invasive Treatment

Surgery

Surgery is the last resort to repair your Achilles tendon.

TREATMENTS FOR ACHILLES TENDON INJURY IN TRADITIONAL CHINESE MEDICINE

Acupuncture

Treatment with acupuncture can bring blood flow to the Achilles tendon and help with the healing.

The main acupuncture points are divided into local and distal points.

Local points are UB 60 Kun Lun, UB 61 Pu Shen, Ki 13 Tai Xi, Ki 14 Da Zhong, Ki 5, Shui Quan and Arshi points around the achilles tendon. *Distal points* are Sp 9 Yin Ling Quan, GB 34 Yang Ling Quan, LI 4 He Gu, and LI 11 Qu Chi (see Table 39.1 and Figure 39.5).

Table 39.1

	Points	Meridian/ Number	Location	Conditions Helped
1	Kun Lun	UB 60	In the depression between the external malleolus and Achilles tendon	Headaches, blurring of vision, neck rigidity, nosebleeds, pain in the shoulder, back, and arm, swelling and pain in the heel, difficult labor, epilepsy
2	Pu Shen	UB 61	In the depression directly below the external malleolus	Epilepsy, mania, headaches, dizziness, insomnia, backache, aching leg
3	Tai Xi	Ki 3	In the depression between the medial malleolus and tendo calcaneus at the level with the tip of the medial malleolus	Sore throat, toothache, deafness, tinnitus, dizziness, spitting of blood, asthma, thirst, irregular menstruation, insomnia, nocturnal emissions, impotence, urinary frequency, lower back pain
4	Da Zhong	Ki 4	Posterior and inferior to the medial malleolus, in the depression medial to the attachment of tendo calcaneus	Spitting of blood, asthma, stiffness and pain of the lower back, painful urination, constipation, pain in the heel, dementia

(Continued)

Table 39.1 (*Continued*)

	Points	Meridian/ Number	Location	Conditions Helped
5	Shui Quan	Ki 5	1 inch directly below Ki 3 Tai Xi in the depression anterior and superior to the medial side of the tuberosity of the calcaneus	Absence of menstruation, irregular menstruation, prolapse of uterus, painful urination, blurring of vision
6	Ying Ling Quan	Sp 9	On the lower border of the medial condyle of the tibia, in the depression on the medial border of the tibia	Abdominal pain and distension, diarrhea, dysentery, swelling, jaundice, painful urination, bedwetting, urinary incontinence, pain in the external genitalia, pain in the knee
7	Yang Ling Quan	GB 34	In the depression anterior and inferior to the head of the fibula	Paralysis, weakness, numbness, and pain in the knee, beriberi, bitter taste in the mouth, vomiting, jaundice, infantile convulsions
8	He Gu	LI 4	*See* Table 13.1/Figure 13.4.	*See* Table 13.1.
9	Qu Chi	LI 11	*See* Table 14.1/Figure 14.4.	*See* Table 14.1.

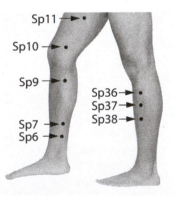

Figure 39.5

ERIC'S TREATMENT

Eric received physical therapy and acupuncture treatment from me for a total of 12 visits. In addition, he stopped doing any sports related to the lower extremities, he regularly put ice on his Achilles tendon, and he walked with wedges in his shoes. The combination of my treatments and the measures I advised him to take on his own succeeded in freeing Eric from the pain his tendonitis had caused, and he was eventually able to resume running.

TIPS FOR PEOPLE WITH AN ACHILLES TENDON INJURY

- Immediately stop your lower extremity exercise, such as running or playing tennis, if you feel pain in the Achilles tendon.
- Put ice on the Achilles tendon and massage it.
- Try to use a heel lift or a shoe wedge to help yourself rest. You may buy one pre-made or go to a shoemaker or an orthotist to have a wedge added to your shoe.
- Never allow anyone to inject steroids into your Achilles tendon because a steroid injection will rupture the tendon.

TIPS FOR ACUPUNCTURE PRACTITIONERS

- Never use a heating pad, lamp, or moxa on the inflamed Achilles tendon, as these will only will increase the inflammation.
- If you suspect a rupture of the Achilles tendon, you must refer the patient to orthopedics.
- Electrical stimulation will help healing.

40

Heel and Foot Pain

Jennifer is a 55-year-old, moderately obese woman. She was in the habit of running about four to five miles every morning, but for two years, she experienced right heel and plantar foot pain, and difficulty walking, especially after waking up in the morning. She went to a podiatrist, who ordered an X-ray that showed a mild spur on her heel. She was given orthotics for the right foot, but she still felt pain, so she came to me for evaluation and treatment.

Upon physical examination, I found a tender point in Jennifer's right heel and arch. There was no ankle pain, and no numbness or tingling sensation in her right leg. Based on my examination and clinical information, I discerned that Jennifer most likely had right plantar fasciitis with a possible heel spur.

SYMPTOMS, CAUSES, AND DIAGNOSIS

There are two different types of plantar foot pain.

Plantar Fasciitis

Plantar fasciitis is inflammation of the thick tissue, called the plantar fascia, on the bottom of the foot. It connects the heel bone to the toes and creates the arch of the foot. The pain is located in your heel and if the pain is severe, it will spread out along the entire foot arch, along the flat band of tissue (ligament) that connects your heel bone to your toes. If you strain your plantar fascia, it gets weak, swollen, and irritated (inflamed). Then your heel or the bottom of your foot hurts when you stand or walk.

The most important, key part, of plantar fasciitis is the overstretched or overused thick band of tissue on the bottom. This can be painful and can make walking or running more difficult. Risk factors for plantar fasciitis include the following.

- Obesity
- High arches and/or flat feet
- Overwalking or running, especially running downhill or on uneven surfaces
- A tight Achilles tendon, the tendon connecting the heel to the calf muscles
- Hard surface of shoes, especially tight and hard shoes without any arch support or cushioning
- Men between the ages of 40 and 70

Heel Spur

A heel spur is a hook of bone that can form on the heel bone (calcaneus). A calcaneal spur (or heel spur) is a radiological (X-ray) finding, and when it is located on the inferior aspect of the calcaneus, it is often associated with plantar fasciitis. However, although some people can have a heel spur without any pain, others can have severe heel pain and that pain can be mixed with plantar fasciitis to cause pain in the entire foot. An inferior calcaneal spur consists of a calcification of bone, which lies above the plantar fascia at the point of its insertion into the heel, most commonly in the medial-side heel of the foot (see Figure 40.1).

Symptoms for both types of plantar heel pain include pain at the bottom of the foot. It is usually sudden onset, most often with a sharp or burning sensation, but sometimes it can be a dull pain.

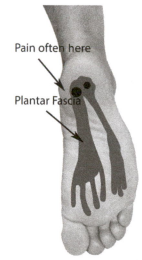

Pain often here

Plantar Fascia

The pain is usually worse in the morning when you take your first steps, after sitting or standing for a while, when climbing stairs or walking on uneven surfaces, or after intense activity.

The pain usually feels better after you warm up or take a hot shower. The pain may develop slowly over time, or arise suddenly after intense activity.

To diagnose plantar problems, the doctor will perform a physical exam that may indicate a tenderness on the bottom of your foot,

Figure 40.1

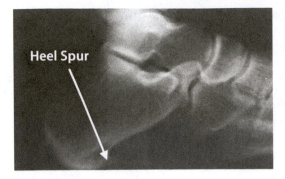

Figure 40.2

usually at the medial heel and entire arch, flat feet or high arches, mild foot swelling or redness, and/or stiffness or tightness of the arch on the bottom of your foot.

X-rays may be taken to rule out other problems, but having a heel spur is a positive finding. (see Figure 40.2).

TREATMENTS FOR HEEL AND FOOT PAIN IN WESTERN MEDICINE

Noninvasive Treatments

Medications

Use acetaminophen (Tylenol) or ibuprofen (Advil, Motrin) to reduce pain and inflammation.

Rest

Rest your foot for at least one week or more, with no running, and no long walks.

Ice

Apply ice to the bottom of your feet for at least 15 minutes, two or three times a day.

Footwear

There are many kinds of footwear used to help plantar fasciitis and heel spurs as shown in the following (see Figures 40.3 to 40.6).

Physical Therapy

Perform a fascia-specific stretching exercise by gently pulling back the toes for 10 sets of 10 seconds each. Repeat three times a day. (See Figure 40.7.)

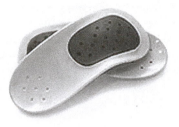

Figure 40.3 Arch support to help with flat feet

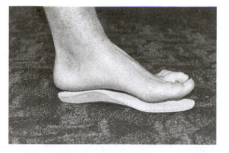

Figure 40.4 Arch support and shoe insole to help with flat feet and plantar fasciitis

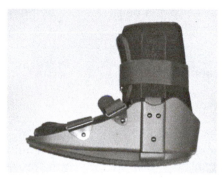

Figure 40.5 Rocker Boot to relieve the pressure of plantar foot and heel

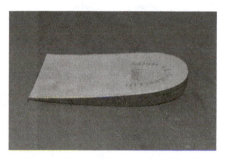

Figure 40.6 Heel pad to relieve the pressure of heel spurs

Put a tennis ball underneath the painful foot and massage it with gradually increased intensity every day, 15–30 minutes each time, two or three times per day. (See Figure 40.8.)

Another exercise targeted at the plantar fascia and good for strengthening the small muscles of the foot is marble pick-ups. Place a handful of marbles

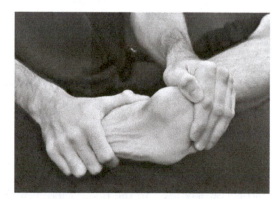

Figure 40.7

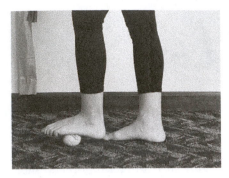

Figure 40.8

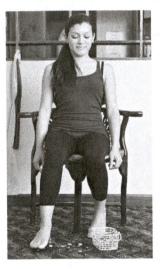

Figure 40.9

on the floor and, using your toes, pick them up and place them in a container. Repeat this for a total of three to five minutes. If marbles are not available, the same motion can be performed using a towel. (See Figure 40.9.)

Ultrasound

The use of the anti-inflammatory properties of ultrasound targeted to the bottom of the heel is beneficial. A typical treatment would last about eight minutes and can be performed by your physical therapist.

Invasive Treatments

Injections

Steroid injections may sometimes make a significant improvement. However, you should use cautiously, because steroids may cause premature death of the cells (necrosis) of the plantar foot.

Surgery

Surgery is the last resort, if all else has failed.

TREATMENTS FOR HEEL AND FOOT PAIN IN TRADITIONAL CHINESE MEDICINE

Acupuncture

The acupuncture points selected are experienced points (Arshi points), Ki 1 Yong Quan, Sp 9 Ying Ling Quan, and GB 34 Yang Ling Quan. The insertion of needles into the plantar foot is a very painful procedure, so the

Table 40.1

	Points	Meridian/ Number	Location	Conditions Helped
1	Arshi Points		Any tender points at the plantar foot; *see* Figure 40.10.	For local pain
2	Yong Quan	Ki 1	On the sole, in the depression when the foot is in plantar flexion, approximately at the junction of the anterior 1/3 and posterior 2/3 of the sole	Headaches, blurring of vision, dizziness, sore throat, dryness of the tongue, loss of voice, painful urination, infantile convulsions, feverish sensation in the sole, loss of consciousness
3	Ying Ling Quan	Sp 9	On the lower border of the medial condyle of the tibia, in the depression on the medial border of the tibia	Abdominal pain and distension, diarrhea, dysentery, swelling, jaundice, painful urination, bedwetting, urinary incontinence, pain in the external genitalia, absence of menstruation, pain in the knee
4	Yang Ling Quan	GB 34	In the depression anterior and inferior to the head of the fibula	Paralysis, weakness, numbness, and pain of the knee, beriberi, bitter taste in the mouth, vomiting, jaundice, infantile convulsions

acupuncturist should choose very tiny, thin needles for the treatment of plantar fasciitis and heel spur (see Figure 40.10 and Table 40.1).

JENNIFER'S TREATMENT

Jennifer was advised to stop running immediately. For treatment, she was given a heel pad with two layers of shoe insoles and changed to

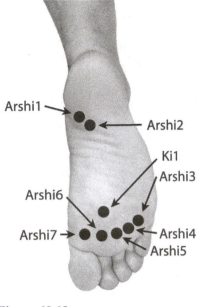

Arshi1
Arshi2
Ki1
Arshi3
Arshi6
Arshi7
Arshi4
Arshi5

Figure 40.10

a larger size of sneakers. She was given the acupuncture treatment outlined earlier and did stretching exercises in physical therapy three times a week for four weeks. Jennifer also stretched her foot on her own and gave herself ice massages three or four times a day. This combination of treatments was very successful. It completely healed her plantar fasciitis, and she was able to run again after two months.

TIPS FOR PEOPLE WITH HEEL AND FOOT PAIN

- Treat the problem early— the earlier, the better.
- Always use two layers of shoe insoles to cushion your inflamed foot.
- Rest and do ice massages.

TIPS FOR ACUPUNCTURE PRACTITIONERS

- Arshi 1 and Arshi 2 are the most important points to reduce plantar pain.
- Use electrical stimulation to desensitize the plantar foot pain.
- Encourage your patients to use shoe insoles. Two layers are better than one layer.
- Try not to use steroid injections.

References

Chapter 1

1. Reston, James, "Now, about My Operation in Peking," *The New York Times*, July 26, 1971.

Chapter 2

1. Melzack R, Wall, PD. "Pain mechanisms: A new theory." *Science*. 150: 171–179, 1965.
2. Wall, PD, Melzack, R. "On the nature of cutaneous sensory mechanisms." *Brain*. 85: 331–356, 1962.
3. Melzack, R. "Acupuncture and pain mechanisms." *Anaesthetist*. 25: 204–207, 1976.
4. Ahsin, S, Saleem, S, Bhatti, AM, et al. "Clinical and endocrinological changes after electro-acupuncture treatment in patients with osteoarthritis of the knee." *Pain*. Sep 17, 2009.
5. Cheng, CH, Yi, PL, Lin, JG, et al. "Endogenous opiates in the nucleus tractus." *Journal of Complementary Alternative Medicine*. Sep 3, 2009.

Chapter 3

1. California Occupational Survey. http://www.acucouncil.org/condi tions_treated.htm
2. WHO. Review and Analysis of Reports on Controlled Clinical Trials. 2003. http://apps.who.int/medicinedocs/en/d/Js4926e/5.html

Chapter 4

1. Acupuncture. NIH. Consensus Statement Online, http://consensus.nih.gov/1997/1997acupuncture107html 15(5): 1–34, Nov 3–5, 1997.

2. Acupuncture: An introduction. National Center for Complementary and Alternative Medicine, NCCAM Publication, No. D404, http://nccam.nih.gov/health/acupuncture/introduction.htm, created December 2007.

3. Melzack R, Wall, PD. "Pain mechanisms: A new theory." *Science.* 150: 171–179, 1965.

4. Wall, PD, Melzack, R. "On the nature of cutaneous sensory mechanism." *Brain.* 85: 331–356, 1962.

5. Melzack, R. "Acupuncture and pain mechanisms." *Anaesthetist.* 25: 204–207, 1976.

6. Silberstein, M. "The cutaneous intrinsic visceral afferent nervous system: A new model for acupuncture analgesia." *Journal of Theoretical Biology.* Sept 15, 2009.

7. Zhang, J, Zhang, N. "Study on mechanisms of acupuncture analgesia." *Zhong Guo Zhen Jiu.* 27(1): 72–75, Jan 2, 2007.

8. Chae, Y, Lee, H, Kim, H, et al. "The neural substrates of verum acupuncture compared to non-penetrating placebo needle: An fMRI study." *Neuroscience Letters.* 450(2): 80–84, Jan 30, 2009.

9. Li, K, Shan B, Xu, J, et al. "Changes in fMRI in the human brain related to different durations of manual acupuncture needling." *Journal of Alternative and Complementary Medicine.* 12(7): 615–623, Sep 13, 2006.

10. Pariente, J, White, P, Frackowiak, RS, et al. "Expectancy and belief modulate the neuronal substrates of pain treated by acupuncture." *Neuroimage.* 25(4): 1161–1167, May 1, 2005.

11. Vickers, AJ, Cronin, AM, et al. "Acupuncture for chronic pain: individual patient data meta-analysis." *Archives of Internal Medicine.* 1–10, Sep 2012.

12. Clark, RJ, Tighe, M, et al. "The effectiveness of acupuncture for plantar heel pain: a systematic review." *Acupuncture in Medicine.* Oct 25, 2012.

13. Macpherson H, Tilbrook H, Bland MJ et al. "Acupuncture for irritable bowel syndrome: Primary care based pragmatic randomized controlled trial." *BMC Gastroenterology.* 12(1): 150, Oct 24, 2012.

14. Cohen, AJ, Menter, A, Hale, L. "Acupuncture: Role in comprehensive cancer care—a primer for the oncologist and review of the literature." *Integrative Cancer Therapies.* (2): 131–143, June 4, 2005.

15. Ezzo, JM, Richardson, MA, Vickers, A, et al. "Acupuncture-point stimulation for chemotherapy-induced nausea or vomiting." *Cochrane Database System Review.* (2): CD002285, Apr 19, 2006.

16. Lee, A, Done, ML. "Stimulation of the wrist acupuncture point P6 for preventing postoperative nausea and vomiting." *Cochrane Database System Review.* 17. CD003281, 2004. Update in: *Cochrane Database System Review.* (2): CD003281, 2009.

17. Yang, CP, Hsieh, CL, et al. "Acupuncture in patients with carpal tunnel syndrome: A randomized controlled trial." *The Clinical Journal of Pain*. (4): 327–33, May 25, 2009.

18. Kumnerddee, W, Kaewtong, A. "Efficacy of acupuncture versus night splinting for carpal tunnel syndrome: A randomized clinical trial." *Journal of the Medical Association of Thailand*. 93(12): 1463–1469, Dec 2010.

19. Cao, L, Zhang, XL, Gao, YS, et al. "Needle acupuncture for osteoarthritis of the knee. A systematic review and updated meta-analysis." *Saudi Medical Journal*. 33(5): 526–532, May 2012.

20. Selfe, TK, Taylor, AG. "Acupuncture and osteoarthritis of the knee: A review of randomized, controlled trials." *Family and Community Health*. 31(3): 247–254, July–Sep 2008.

21. Witt, CM, Jena, S, Brinkhaus, B, et al. "Acupuncture in patients with osteoarthritis of the knee or hip: A randomized, controlled trial with an additional nonrandomized arm." *Arthritis and Rheumatism*. 54(11): 3485–3493, Nov 2006.

22. Sunay, D, Sunay, M, et al. "Acupuncture versus paroxetine for the treatment of premature ejaculation: A randomized, placebo-controlled clinical trial." *European Urology*. 59(5): 765–771, May 2011.

23. Dieterle, S, Li, C, Greb, R, et al. "Prospective randomized placebo-controlled study of the effect of acupuncture in infertile patients with severe oligoasthenozoospermia." *Fertility and Sterility*. 92(4): 1340–1343, Oct 2009.

24. Manheimer, E, Zhang, G, Udoff, L, et al. "Effects of acupuncture on rates of pregnancy and live birth among women undergoing in vitro fertilisation: Systematic review and meta-analysis." *British Medical Journal*. 336(7643): 545–549, Mar 8, 2008.

25. Cho, YJ, Song, YK, et al. "Acupuncture for chronic low back pain: A multicenter, randomized, patient-assessor blind, sham-controlled clinical trial." *Spine*. Sep 28, 2012.

26. Thomas, KJ, MacPherson, H, et al. "Longer term clinical and economic benefits of offering acupuncture care to patients with chronic low back pain." *Health Technology Assessment*. (32): iii–iv, ix–x, 1–109, Aug 9, 2005.

27. Liang, Z, Zhu, X, et al. "Assessment of a traditional acupuncture therapy for chronic neck pain: a pilot randomised controlled study." *Complementary Therapies in Medicine*. 19 (Suppl 1): S26–32, Jan 2011.

28. Molsberger, AF, Schneider, T, et al. "German Randomized Acupuncture Trial for chronic shoulder pain (GRASP)—a pragmatic, controlled, patient-blinded, multi-centre trial in an outpatient care environment." *Pain*. 151(1): 146–154, Oct 2010.

Chapter 6

1. Lai, X, Xu, N. *The Guidelines of Acupuncture and Clinical Research*. Beijing, 2008. www.sciencep.com

Chapter 11

1. Website: http://www.allergan.com/treatments/neurosciences/cervical_ dystonia.htm#fn2

2. Website: http://www.allergan.com/treatments/neurosciences/cervical_ dystonia.htm#fn2

3. Website: http://www.wihrd.soton.ac.uk/projx/signpost/steers/STEER_ 2002%2810%29.pdf

Chapter 29

1. Turner, J, et al. "Surgery for lumbar spinal stenosis. Attempted meta-analysis of the literature." *Spine*. 17: 1–8, 1992.

Chapter 30

1. Websites: http://www.biomedcentral.com/1471–2474/7/92/ http:// www.ncbi.nlm.nih.gov/pubmed/15040822?dopt=AbstractPlus

2. Xu, J. *Magic Needles: Feel Younger and Live Longer with Acupuncture.* Laguna Beach, CA: Basic Health Publications, Inc., 2011, p. 208.

Chapter 35

1. Lussier, A, Cividino, AA, McFarlane, CA, et al. "Viscosupplementation with Hylan for the treatment of osteoarthritis: Findings from clinical practice in Canada." *Journal of Rheumatology*. 23: 1579–1585, 1996.

2. Selfe, TK, Taylor, AG. "Acupuncture and osteoarthritis of the knee: A review of randomized, controlled trials." *Family & Community Health*. 31(3): 247–254, July–Sep 2008.

Chapter 39

1. Ahmed, IM, Lagopoulos, M, McConnell, P, et al. Department of Human Biology, University of Leeds, England. "Blood supply of the Achilles tendon." *Journal of Orthopaedic Research*. 16(5): 591–596, Sep 1998.

Resources

Chinese Acupuncture and Moxibustion. Editor in Chief, Cheng Xinnong, Beijing Foreign Languages Press, 1987.

Chinese Acupuncture Prescription Collection. Editor in Chief, Wang Lizhao, Jiangxi Scientific and Technology Press, 1990.

Miraculous Skills in Traditional Chinese Acupuncture and Moxibustion. Editor in Chief, Shi Xue-Min, Tianjin Scientific and Translation Press, 1992.

Index

Abdominal pain, 10
Abductor pollicis longus, 123
ACAOM. *See* Accreditation Commission for Acupuncture and Oriental Medicine
Accreditation Commission for Acupuncture and Oriental Medicine (ACAOM), 21
Achilles tendon injury: diagnosis of, 280–81; physical therapy for, 281–82; points for, 283–84; surgery for, 282; symptoms of, 279–81; TCM treatments for, 283–85; treatment tips for, 285; Western medical treatments for, 281–82
Acne vulgaris, 10
Acromioclavicular joint, 112
Acromioclavicular spur, 110
Acupuncture: ACAOM, 21; balance systems in, 24–25; California State Committee Survey for, 8–11; committees/surveys about, 7–10; conditions worth trying, 11; contemporary model for, 14; cultural growth of, 13; current Chinese theories of, 23–25; diseases commonly treated by, 3, 8–9; Eastern explanation of, 6; endorphins affected by, 24; history

of, 3–5; *Magic Needles-Feel Younger and Live Longer with Acupuncture* (XU), 300; Maryland Society of, 9; NCCAOM, 21, 299; reactions to, 22; recent research conditions suitable for, 14–19; state licensing for, 21; Western explanation of, 6–7; WHO expert report on, 9–11. *See also* Points; Traditional Chinese medicine
Acupuncturists: MD, 20–21, 299–300; non-physician, 21–22
Acute Achilles tendonitis, 281
Acute low back sprain: bed rest for, 158; lumbosacral brace for, 158–59; medications for, 158; physical therapy for, 159; points for, 160–61; symptoms/causes/diagnosis of, 157–58; TCM treatments for, 159–62
Acute neck spasms: points for, 93–95; symptoms/causes/diagnosis of, 92; TCM treatments for, 93–96; treatment tips for, 96; Western medical treatments for, 93
Adhesive capsulitis. *See* Frozen shoulder
Albert Einstein College of Medicine, 299
Alcohol dependence, 10

About the Author

Dr. Jun Xu is a medical doctor in Connecticut specializing in rehabilitative medicine and acupuncture in his private practice. He is an attending physician and acupuncturist in the Department of Medicine of Stamford Hospital in Connecticut and is also an assistant professor in the Department of Rehabilitation Medicine of the New York Medical College in New York City.

Xu spent eight years training in traditional Chinese medicine (TCM) and acupuncture and received his medical degree and master of medicine from two medical schools in China. He then taught and practiced medicine and acupuncture at Guangzhou College of Chinese Medicine in China.

In the 1980s, Xu migrated to America, and became a postdoctoral research fellow, first at the University of Georgia and then at Albert Einstein College of Medicine in the Bronx, New York. He interned for a year at the St. Francis Medical Center of the University of Pittsburgh Medical School, Pittsburgh, Pennsylvania, and then transferred to the New York Medical College, where he received his three-year resident training in physical medicine and rehabilitation. After graduation, he started his private practice in both physical medicine and acupuncture.

Dr. Xu is certified by the American Board of Physical Medicine and Rehabilitation. He is a diplomat in acupuncture and Chinese herbology, certified by the National Commission for the Certification of Acupuncture and Oriental Medicine, and has acupuncture and MD physician licenses in several states, including Connecticut.

Dr. Xu's medical society memberships include the American Academy of Physical Medicine and Rehabilitation and the Association of Chinese American Physicians. Between March 2010 and March 2012, he served as president of the American Traditional Chinese Medicine Society, where he had previously served as vice president.

This is the author's second book on the subject of acupuncture. The first, Magic Needles—Feel Younger and Live Longer with Acupuncture, was published in 2011 to wide acclaim and, although written to appeal to a general audience, as is this book, it has become a resource for medical students and acupuncture practitioners wishing to have a superior knowledge of this ancient, highly effective Chinese method of treatment.

Dr. Xu has been featured in magazines and on several television shows, including Good Morning America, News Channel 12 in Norwalk, CT, and The Greenwich Times in Greenwich, Connecticut. In addition, he has lectured and has published a significant number of research articles for medical journals. He lives in Scarsdale, New York, with his wife and children.

More information about Dr. Xu can be found at http://drxuacupuncture.com/.